# The Dog and I

# The Dog and I

## CONFESSIONS OF A BEST FRIEND

Roy MacGregor

VIKING
CANADA

VIKING CANADA

Published by the Penguin Group

Penguin Group (Canada), 90 Eglinton Avenue East, Suite 700, Toronto, Ontario, Canada M4P 2Y3
    (a division of Pearson Canada Inc.)

Penguin Group (USA) Inc., 375 Hudson Street, New York, New York 10014, U.S.A.
Penguin Books Ltd, 80 Strand, London WC2R 0RL, England
Penguin Ireland, 25 St Stephen's Green, Dublin 2, Ireland (a division of Penguin Books Ltd)
Penguin Group (Australia), 250 Camberwell Road, Camberwell, Victoria 3124, Australia
    (a division of Pearson Australia Group Pty Ltd)
Penguin Books India Pvt Ltd, 11 Community Centre, Panchsheel Park, New Delhi – 110 017, India
Penguin Group (NZ), cnr Airborne and Rosedale Roads, Albany, Auckland 1310, New Zealand
    (a division of Pearson New Zealand Ltd)
Penguin Books (South Africa) (Pty) Ltd, 24 Sturdee Avenue, Rosebank, Johannesburg 2196, South Africa

Penguin Books Ltd, Registered Offices: 80 Strand, London WC2R 0RL, England

First published 2006

(RRD)   10 9 8 7 6 5 4 3 2 1

Manufactured in Canada.

ISBN-10:  0-670-06554-4
ISBN-13:  978-0-670-06554-7

Library and Archives Canada Cataloguing in Publication available upon request.

Visit the Penguin Group (Canada) website at **www.penguin.ca**

Special and corporate bulk purchase rates available; please see
**www.penguin.ca/corporatesales** or call 1-800-399-6858, ext. 477 or 474

*In appreciation of Buddy, Cindy, Bumps, Bandit, Cricket,*
*and Willow, who have made our lives so much richer*

# Contents

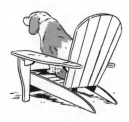

## Extreme Youth

# Alleged Adulthood

# So Very Old

# Introduction

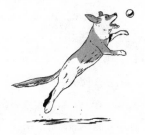

*"No!"* I said. *"Drop it!"*

Sad to say, dogs are much better than daughters when it comes to obeying simple commands. She wasn't listening.

Our old mutt, Bandit, had not long before moved on to wherever it is that old dogs go when everything gives out, from eyes to ears to back end. It had reached the point, finally, where even the adult human in absolute denial had to act, and sadly, we did.

With Bandit so recently departed, I had no interest at

all in a puppy crossing the front-door threshold—fully aware of the consequences.

Once a puppy makes it through that front door, it's in.

That's just the way it is with puppies and front doors. Imagine, if you can, a parent watching his or her partner come through the door with their brand-new baby, which the waiting parent then holds up to check the heft and colouring and sex before handing the infant back with a dismissive "Not this one, thanks—let's have a look at another."

So no puppy; at least not yet.

Yes, it was difficult coming home from a long road trip and not having that one member of the family who isn't shouting "What did you bring me?" race to greet you. And yes, it was odd getting up each morning and going to bed each night without opening the sliding doors that lead to the backyard so that Bandit could go through all the necessary sniffing and squatting and barking at various territorial invaders before closing off her day. But still, I wasn't ready.

Jocelyn wouldn't listen though. Our daughter was already surfing the net in search of something that might approximate the glorious mutt we had just lost. She was poring through shelter listings, checking out Humane Societies within a three-hour driving range, and letting everyone know that someone who needs a dog doesn't yet have one.

No ... no ... *NO!* she was told.

She interpreted that to mean "Yes" and, I must confess, that may be exactly what it was. A "yes" with trepidation.

So when I saw Jocelyn pull into the driveway after a long weekend up in the Ottawa Valley I cannot today say if I was pleased or disappointed that I could see no basket, no wagging tail, no furry little head staring over an elbow at the new world it was about to take over.

There was really no time to think one way or the other. She ran up the steps, through the door, and simply unfurled her jacket to release a little white and yellow furball that hit the floor wiggling and wagging and hasn't stopped wiggling or wagging in the year since.

The new puppy was in.
And in to stay.

"I COULD TELL YOU the story of my life through the dogs I have loved," Erica Jong once wrote in an essay trying to explain her preference for the canine world over the human. "I could tell you the story of the losses in my life through their deaths. Dogs come into our lives to teach us about love and loyalty. They depart to teach us about loss. We try to replace them but never quite succeed. A new dog never replaces an old dog; it merely expands the heart."

I am now on to my fifth dog, though that seems a foolish way to put it; nothing seems as crass as treating a dog as you would an appliance that needs replacing from time to time. Better to say, as Erica Jong suggests, that I have fallen in love again. This time with Willow, a floppy-eared little mutt with long white and tan hair as soft as down, a face sharp as a fox, and a weakness for carrying around dirty socks in her mouth.

I think I was born a dog person; it just took a while to become one. When I was very young we lived part of each year in Ontario's vast Algonquin Park, and dogs—especially deer-chasing dogs—were discouraged by those who were there to protect the wildlife. My grandfather was chief ranger; and while he too loved dogs, it wouldn't do for the head man to have one running around when no one else did.

I was eleven when I was finally able to have a puppy, though it was made clear that Buddy would have to be tied up whenever we were staying at the grandparents' log home on Lake of Two Rivers. That sweet little puppy never got to become a dog, but he still leads the list of "dogs I have loved."

Buddy came from a rundown house down by the Muskoka River. A kid who, like me, had a *Toronto Daily Star* paper route also had a litter of part-shepherd, part-hound, part-guess puppies to dispose of, and one late-winter afternoon I picked out a little male, free of charge, and carried him back up Reservoir Hill to where we lived.

Then came Cindy, a half cocker spaniel with a tail so active it couldn't possibly be bobbed, at a cost of three dollars from a house on the edge of town. Cindy overlapped slightly with Bumps, the first of what we would come to call "borderline collies," a soft little black and white puppy that came from across the street when we lived in Toronto and cost not a cent. Bumps was followed by Bandit, a ten-dollar mutt, part border collie, part Lab, from a village down along the Rideau River. And now, thanks to Jocelyn's inability to obey simple commands, there is Willow, part border collie, part puzzle from higher up the Ottawa River at Petawawa, cost one hundred dollars, but that included shots.

So let's add it all up. Five dogs—three of whom lived to sixteen—spanning forty-six years at a total initial investment of $113. That works out to $2.45 a year.

The price of a coffee and doughnut to get you through the morning.

Or the cost of a faithful companion to get you through life.

IT'S BEEN ABOUT TWENTY YEARS since I began writing a daily newspaper column for the *Ottawa Citizen*. I took on this new job with great seriousness and, at times, would work for hours interviewing and researching and thinking before sitting down to write the definitive piece on a politician or a compelling social problem.

Most days, such columns passed without comment. In a way, that is actually good news to those of us who work in the daily newspaper industry, as feedback usually tilts to the critical. Those who agree with you tend to nod; those who disagree write; those who *really* disagree write your boss.

The day I wrote my very first dog column, I wondered if I dare. People have dogs, and people talk about their dogs, but were dogs a suitable topic for a self-styled serious columnist? Was the subject too light? Too insignificant? Was I wasting valuable news space? I went ahead anyway—and was overwhelmed by the response.

And since then, every time I have wondered if I should write about the dog, I have been shocked the next day that I even cautioned for a moment.

Some of those columns, largely abridged, are included here, but more than half of the material is original, specifically written for this book that first began to take shape more than a year ago. There are columns and small essays on the joy of puppies, the trials of the teenage dog, the pleasures of the mature dog and, of course, the heartbreak of the dog lost. Four of those fine friends—Buddy, Cindy, Bumps, and Bandit—are no longer with us.

Or so the saying goes.

In fact, they are always with us.

There might be books about humans teaching dogs, but they have it somewhat backwards.

# It's a
# Dog's Life

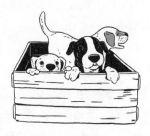

I once had a dog who purred.

I was eleven years old when I got Cindy. She was not my first dog, but became the first to span a significant amount of my own life—childhood, teen years, school years, marriage, right up to within months of first child.

The actual first dog, Buddy, was a small black and white mutt with fur as soft as rabbit. Sadly, he never had a chance to lose that puppy fur. I was at school when my mother let him out the back door to pee and he bolted on her. We lived on Reservoir Hill in the small Ontario town of Huntsville, on a street so steep cars couldn't get up it most winter days, and the frisky little puppy ran right out onto the road just as the garbage truck happened to be thundering down the hill and couldn't be stopped quickly by anything short of a row of maple trees. Buddy was killed instantly.

I never even got to say goodbye because my mother, a practical person who did indeed have a good heart, agreed with the garbagemen that they could best dispose of the body. The driver felt bad. My mother felt terrible. I, of course, was devastated and, for years after—in fact, for decades after—would have recurring dreams that little Buddy, his fur still soft as satin, had found his way back to the door where she had let him out and was scratching to get in.

A few months after Buddy's loss, not long after the first snow that year, a small advertisement appeared in the back pages of the *Huntsville Forester:*

> *Puppies for Sale*
> *Mixed breed, mother spaniel, $3*

There was a telephone number included, and I talked my mother into at least calling to see if they were all gone. She did and they weren't. There were three puppies left, but they were "going fast."

I do not think she believed that. Puppies, in those years, were not something you sold. They were simply available, handed out by kids carrying a wagonload of squealing puppies around the neighbourhood or "advertised" by a crude sign hanging at the end of a farm lane that said, simply, "Puppies," or, though additional information wasn't really necessary, "Free Puppies." My mother wasn't at all impressed by the cost and clearly thought that asking for money was bad form.

I have tried to understand how things could change so drastically. Looking back all those years, it seems that purebreds and papers and thousand-dollar dogs were something that must have come along later, like second cars and microwaves and plasma-screen televisions. I do remember one huge dog up the street. Bo Bo must have been mostly a German shepherd, but was as close to royal lines as the town got—belonging to a family in the logging business and, by extension, virtual monarchy in this little town that then depended on the timber trade.

Dogs were mutts, though no one ever used that name because all dogs were mutts. The dog next door, Buster, was a mutt. The dog across the street, a cranky little thing called Jiggs, was a mutt. The dog two doors down, Lady, was a mutt. Four doors down, Queenie, a mutt. None, of course, looked at all the same as another; but none, as well, looked at all the same as any other dog in town—unless, of course, they happened to come from the same litter. But even then you couldn't count on it.

Somehow, I talked my mother into letting me go out to this place. I had money from my *Toronto Daily Star* paper route, so I put together three bucks in change and jammed it into the pocket of my big sweater. My mother was a great knitter—a famous knitter, in fact, for the area—and brought in extra money by knitting big wool sweaters that she sold for the cost of the wool and about fifteen cents an hour for labour. She knit sweaters with white-tailed deer on the back; big, bulky sweaters with pheasants; sweaters with moose, bears, eagles, wolves; sweaters with hunters and hockey players. Mine, of course, was a hockey player.

The sweater was thick and warm and I put it on for the long walk out to the edge of town. It was a very long walk—we had no car at all, let alone a second car—and the journey, in lightly blowing snow, took me up Main Street, out along the railroad tracks and the choppy, steel-coloured bay that had yet to freeze over, and close enough to the edge of town that you could see and hear the lumber trucks thundering past on the new Highway 11 bypass.

There, across from a small planing mill, was a red brick bungalow. I knocked at the door and waited, fidgeting.

A woman came to the door. She was dark and severe and was wearing a purple housecoat and smoking a cigarette. The room inside was also purple, with smoke. The cigarette, which stayed in her painted mouth, looked as though it had been bleeding about the filter.

"Yes?" she said. No hello, no greeting.

I was used to meeting people at their front door. I had to collect every two weeks for my *Star* route.

"Is this the place with the puppies?" I asked.

She nodded, two thick parallel streams of smoke coming out her nostrils. "They cost three dollars," she said, expecting that to be the end of the conversation.

"I have it," I said, grabbing my sweater pocket and shaking the change.

She opened the door and stepped aside. "They're in the basement."

I went in, took off my rubber boots—black, the kind we rolled down as low as we could so that the white insides hung over them like a cape and rendered the boots essentially useless for what they were made for—and trailed after her in thick grey woollen socks desperately in need of pulling up.

She led the way, opening a door off the kitchen and stepping gingerly down a couple of steps while she searched along the rough framing for the light switch. She found it and we both went down, I amazed at how clear and clean the air was, she coughing impatiently.

A blond spaniel was there, somewhat cowering, bobbed tail wagging. Her nipples were almost dragging on the cement floor as she waddled across from a basket and crouched in front of the woman with the cigarette.

In the basket were three small furballs.

"You can have your pick," she said.

There may be no tougher decision in life. It is easier to decide on a job than a puppy, easier to pick out a new car than a new dog.

One was dark brown with black spots. One was black with brown spots. Both of these were male. The third was almost the spitting image of the mother. She had silky, curly blond hair and a small face that held the biggest, saddest brown eyes I had ever seen in my life.

She was also the only girl—something I hadn't figured on. Like most stupid humans, I had always thought of dogs as male and cats as female, even though an eleven-year-old is perfectly aware that one of each is necessary to produce more of each.

I picked them up one by one and turned them over, the little things biting at my hands with razor teeth, their little tails whipping. The males were cute, and aggressive, but the little female was ... *beautiful*.

I was instantly in love. "I guess I'll take this one," I said. There was no *guess* about it. The dog had already decided.

"They're weaned," the woman said, "but maybe you should feed her some cream for a bit."

I nodded, but I wasn't really listening. I was staring at this beautiful, tiny little creature that lay upside down in my cupped hands. I was holding her like a communion wafer (that winter I'd started serving in the Anglican church down by the river). It seemed oddly appropriate.

I fished out the change. She counted it, nodded, and put it into the pocket of her housecoat. She turned and began going up the stairs.

The other puppies were whining and squealing. I wondered if they knew their sister was leaving. Perhaps they were just hungry. The woman, however, paid them no attention at all.

She showed me—*us*—to the door, did not even reach out to pat the little puppy she would never see again, but suddenly showed her first genuine concern for the dogs. "Keep her warm," she said. "It's getting cold out there."

It was freezing now. Much colder than when I'd started out. The wind cut through the sweater as if it were nothing but holes—which, of course, it was, even if tightly packed. It was also beginning to darken. I'd barely have time to get her home before I'd have to head off to collect and deliver my papers. This was when most newspapers were still afternoon events, something people read at leisure in the evening rather than in panic in the morning.

The wind was now coming hard straight off the bay. It had turned into a day where it is somehow easier to walk backwards than forwards, so I did, switching every now and then to check my bearings.

I carried her for a while in the pocket of the sweater, the same pocket that had held the change. I have never forgotten the sensation of that moment all these years later, the strange feeling of walking along with a live dog in my pocket. A dog so small that no one passing by in the cars and trucks would ever even notice. A dog that was wiggling and twisting so much that I had to keep a mitt over the pocket to make sure she didn't suddenly pop out like a jack-in-the-box that has triggered its own lid.

After a while I moved her from the pocket to inside the big sweater and then inside the second sweater. I folded my arms over my stomach as if I had a bellyache, she spread herself long and tight along my body heat, and I hurried faster to get her home.

I still had her there when I came into the house. My glasses were steaming up so fast I knew they wouldn't clear for several minutes, so I just tossed them onto the kitchen table. My mother was at the stove. I folded up the two layers of sweater, pulled her out, set her down, and watched, in shock, as she first peed and then pooped on the kitchen floor.

Any who doubted my mother's heart earlier cannot doubt it now. She said not a word. She cleaned it up herself and then took the little dog in her hands and checked it over as if it were something she'd picked up at the A&P produce counter. She checked the legs, the ears, the stomach, the teeth.

"You know it's a girl?" she said.

"Yessss," I said, as if she had just asked the most obvious question possible.

"We'll have to have her spayed," she said.

I nodded. I wasn't quite sure about all this. I knew it meant no puppies, and that was fine by me. But I hadn't anticipated the whole extent of the problem.

"It costs a lot of money," she said. "And we'll have to take her to Bracebridge to have it done."

There was no veterinarian in our little town. Instantly, I was thrown into a pickle. We'd need transportation to get her to Bracebridge. We'd have to leave her and would need transportation to get her back. And we'd need money to pay for the operation.

Males, on the other hand, need no such thing. Once the three dollars had been paid, that would have been it for a male.

My mother smiled. "But she sure is cute."

NAMING A DOG is almost as hard as taking the pick of the litter. For days I'd been searching for the perfect name for this little blond puppy, and while dozens of names had been written down on a sheet of paper, only to be scratched out after a few practice throws, I'd more or less settled on one that seemed, to me, to fit.

"She's 'Bridget,'" I told my grandmother once I'd carried the little thing down the street and up the stairs to her small apartment closer to Main Street.

*"What?"* she snapped.

This reaction completely caught me by surprise. My grandmother was a woman normally of great good humour, but she had the Irish temperament and could be a most formidable force. Not much over five feet tall, she had for decades ruled, with absolute power, a home where her husband had long been the towering chief ranger of the local provincial park. But even in full uniform he was at all times acutely aware of who was the true commanding officer.

Being afraid of her fury was hardly restricted to the family. My two brothers and sister once watched in awe as a huge black bear came sniffing down the trail behind their log home on Lake of Two Rivers. She had been baking in the kitchen, and when she saw the bear coming closer she grabbed the broom and raced out so fast that the screen door hadn't even slammed when the bear suddenly halted dead in its tracks at the sight of this little pepper pot coming straight at him in full attack mode, broom swinging as she shouted, *"GET OUTTA HERE, YOU!"*

The bear spun and bolted back up the trail so fast that, to this day (a half century on), my siblings and I are convinced his back legs outran his front, virtually turning him inside out as he crashed into the spruce cover and safety.

"Bridget," I repeated.

"That's no name for a dog," she said. No, she *ordered*.

I had thought it perfect. I'm not sure today where it came from, but it may have had to do with the curling blond hair on the dog and Brigitte Bardot, whose very name then was somehow held to be equivalent to a dirty joke. So now I thought, naturally, that this is what must be bothering her. You couldn't call your dog Brigitte Bardot in good company.

"You'll have to find something else," she commanded.

Eventually we did—compromising on "Cindy," though I have no recollection at all where that came from.

For nearly forty years I never thought again of "Bridget"—not until a distant cousin began digging through the roots of the family tree. He had been searching through church records of the Upper Ottawa Valley. Both sides of the family—Scots and Irish on my father's, pure Irish on my mother's—had come to the Valley in the days before and during the various potato famines of the 1840s. Apart from a large and unwieldy family Bible that held a few birth records, wedding registries, and haphazard notes, not much was known about those early years and, truth be told, no one had much cared before this relative's sudden interest in genealogy.

When he could not find the birth records he was seeking in the Anglican church of the town of Renfrew, he switched over to the other Protestant churches and, finally, to the Catholic church. And here he uncovered an astonishing family secret.

My grandmother, listed in the old family Bible as Bea Dowd—my sister, Ann, had even been given the middle name "Beatrice" in honour of her—had been born Catholic, baptized "Bridget O'Dowd" and, somewhere along the line, dropped both her name and her church before she married Tom McCormick, a Protestant from a farm near the little Ottawa Valley village of Antrim.

In the Valley in those days, Protestants and Catholics were often bitter enemies—my father often telling us how the Catholic kids and the Protestant kids of Eganville would gather on their church sides of the Bonnechere River that split the town and hurl rocks at each other.

No wonder she had recoiled so much at my naming the dog "Bridget." The name was never heard again. We called her "Cindy"—and eventually she even came to it.

IN A WAY we grew up together. Since I was eleven when I got her, we were teenagers together, and there's no doubt, looking back, that she reached maturity far sooner than I did.

She was middle-aged when I headed off to school in a city several hours to the north and, from then on, I would be home only infrequently. She, of course, was home constantly. My mother, who had fed her since that first day I carried the three-dollar puppy home in my sweater pocket, took on the care of the dog. She fed her, let her in and out, and even put up a plywood barrier into the back room so that Cindy could be in and warm in winter, but come the good weather she was out day and night.

My mother believed, as so many of her generation did, that dogs were meant to be kept outside as much as possible. She had a good doghouse built by a local handyman and put in some burlap sacks for comfort. She hooked up a chain to a clothesline so that Cindy could get some exercise. The dog, however, was now much older, going on ten, and hardly needed what was once necessary.

The problem was not my mother and not the dog. The problem was the owner, and it is a common story among humans and dogs. The kid who once could hardly think of anything but hanging out with his dog became a teenager and wanted to hang out with a different crowd. He failed at school. He dropped out of sports. He fell for a local girl and forgot completely about the old dog. The girl's father was a teacher and, out of necessity, the boy recovered at school, if only barely, and then moved away to go to a higher school. He was too busy for an old dog—even one who would still go crazy the second she saw him and moan and groan and almost hum if only he could spare a few moments of his frightfully busy and important life to scratch her belly.

I know there is nothing particularly new in this because I have heard it from others. It doesn't, however, make it any more acceptable.

A friend of mine, a lovely writer named Bob Levin, once put into words the regret and guilt felt by those who have a lifelong companion they forget to make time for. Bob's dog was also a mutt, named Rock, and he wrote about his feelings in a powerful piece that appeared in the *Toronto Star* late in 2005. His feelings of remorse, and his sense that he had to deal with them, came back to him when, of all things, he was watching a television newscast of the flooding that hit New Orleans following Hurricane Katrina. The dogs on the rooftops and out on the tree limbs reminded him of Rock in the way that they simply stared at those people far too busy filming to help them—a stare that said, simply, "I deserve better."

Bob had grown up in the United States but his story of regret was shockingly similar. Rock had come from the Humane Society in Philadelphia and had been a bit of a wonder dog, smart and affectionate, part pointer, part mystery. The two were inseparable. She was stubborn but equally loyal, and had every right to expect such dedication returned.

The years went by and, of course, he went off, first to college, then into an increasingly successful magazine career. As his life became busier and busier, Rock eventually got slower and slower. She had bladder problems; they lived in a fourth-floor New York apartment and, when accidents happened, he let his irritation show.

Then Rock reached fifteen and began having heart problems.

Here is how Bob described the moment when he realized he'd failed her:

> *I can't recall what was bugging me that day; I like*
> *to think there was something. But as we walked*
> *toward the car, she just stopped, wouldn't budge.*
> *I told her to come on and, when she still wouldn't,*
> *I yelled and yanked her leash—hard—and that's*
> *when she flashed me the look.*
>
> *I'm not that stubborn, the look said. I just can't*
> *move. I don't deserve this.*

She didn't and he knew it. Bob felt that his impatience and self-absorption had somehow led to what he could only call "the betrayal of a dear friend." He knelt, hugged the old dog, and says that her heart was pounding so hard it almost flew out of her chest. A few days later the old heart gave out completely. He happened to be at work when word came, and he went into his boss's office and told her and this woman had the sense and compassion to come around her desk and hug him while they both cried. Dog lovers will understand.

My betrayal of Cindy took other routes. I became self-absorbed and then absorbed with another human whom I eventually married. We moved away to the city, two hours plus by car; and, though we returned often, there seemed barely time for a pat on the head before we were off swimming or skiing.

A quick pat and a quick hard scratch around the ears— Cindy always moaning in delight, no matter how long it lasted—and that was about it. Since she was now too old to run and keep up, she was rarely taken, rarely even considered.

Besides, there was a new model and she could not compete. We lived in a bit of a lower-class area of Toronto and the kids across the street came around one day asking if anyone would like a puppy. They had a litter of seven—lineage known only so far as the father appeared to be the black and white beast from down the street and the mother was obviously the part terrier nursing the little creatures—and they simply wanted to give them away. Free of charge. Just like in the old days.

Ellen picked out a small black and white one that looked like the suspected father, a border collie. She named her "Bumps" after a nickname her sister, Jacqueline, had picked up years earlier as a falling-down toddler and had gradually shaken off. So it was free to be used again in the family.

Bumps went everywhere with us. She swam and skied. Once she was house-trained, she slept on the bed and lay on the furniture and drove in the passenger's side of the second-hand Datsun we eventually purchased. New lifestyle. New (sort of) car. New dog.

Life could not be better—unless your name was Cindy.

My moment of realization came as a shocker. Cindy had had such little exercise—doghouse to dish, dish to doghouse, run the line to the end of the yard, run back, her feet never touching pavement or rough ground— that her toenails grew so long they began to curl back in on her. A bloodied paw and a race to the vet—there finally being one in town—changed everything.

Ellen suggested we take the old dog back to Toronto with us. The old dog needed more exercise, if only to keep her toenails worn down on pavement and concrete. Besides, Ellen argued, the two dogs would be good company for each other when we were at work. Cindy got along wonderfully with the puppy, even if every once in a while she had to snap at Bumps to keep the puppy in line or bowl her over just to show that there was not *total* indulgence going on here.

It made sense, even though I must admit the thought had never occurred to me. In those days, I will now admit, not many thoughts occurred to me.

We took her back to the city with us, a twelve-year-old sort-of-spaniel along with a less-than-year-old kind-of border collie, though it was hard on the ride down to tell which was the puppy and which the grizzled old dog. Cindy prowled the back seat, pushed to get into the front and, finally, sat staring out the back window much as any northern bush hick on a first trip to the big city.

I never expected to get four years out of her. She outlasted the car. She outlasted a second car.

Twice a day, sometimes more, she was taken for long, long walks around the neighbourhood and down into the nearby ravine. She became a favourite of the kids for the way she would groan and moan contentedly as they scratched her ears.

"She purrs," Grace, one of the neighbourhood kids who had brought us Bumps, said one day.

We smiled. She did indeed purr.

We took her out west that second summer, Cindy and Bumps with the run of the back seat in that brief period before the children started to come as fast as puppies.

She took her obligations as older dog seriously. If Bumps was too frisky, she was put in her place. If Bumps tried to sneak a closer place in our bed, she was soon sent back while Cindy snuggled in and began to ... purr.

Her intelligence never dimmed. While out West we went hiking along the steep hills of the Qu'Appelle Valley near Ellen's family's Saskatchewan farm. Bumps, ever too anxious, would tumble down the hills, slipping, falling, and making a fool of herself until Cindy came along and promptly rounded her up with a few sharp snips. She then carefully showed Bumps the dog secret to steep hills, to walk them as switchbacks, *tacking,* as it were, down the hill against the grade. It was a lesson Bumps never forgot.

I never forgot my lesson, either. That neglect—that abandonment, that *betrayal*—could have haunted me forever had not Ellen repaired the damage. It wasn't just the paw that was bleeding.

Cindy had the best four years of her life with us. She remained healthy and well right up until Ellen became very pregnant with our first, and then it was almost as if she decided to make way.

We were walking her and Bumps in deep snow down through the ravine. It was a bright, cold day, a perfect day for dog walking, when suddenly Ellen said, "There's something wrong with Cindy."

There was indeed. She was shaking her head as if blackflies were in her ears, but that, of course, was impossible. She was stumbling as she walked. We went and knelt with her, holding her. Just as with Bob Levin's Rock, Cindy's heart was pounding. She was frightened, confused. She could not hold her balance. Her one eye seemed ... dead.

"I think she's had a stroke," Ellen said.

I nodded, unable to say anything.

We carried her home, wrapped her in blankets, and called the veterinarian's office. It was just up the street so we hurried in, an emergency. The vet—a wonderfully patient man with the best bedside manners I've ever seen—confirmed the suspicion. A stroke. And a serious one. He talked to us for a long while about quality of life. He didn't have to. This is what this whole thing had been about for the last four years.

He said she was suffering and would suffer even more if we did not act out of compassion. He did not suggest but we took up the suggestion anyway. We would do it right away. He asked if we wished to be with her. Of course we did.

He gave us a few minutes alone with her. There were tears, of course, though none from her. She was periodically wagging her tail and looking up with the one eye that still seemed as though it could see.

"Ready?" he asked, opening the door only slightly.

We opened it the rest of the way. "Ready." But, of course, we weren't. No one ever is for what it feels like.

It was very quick, very quiet. Ellen stroked Cindy's head as the needle went in.

And Cindy purred.

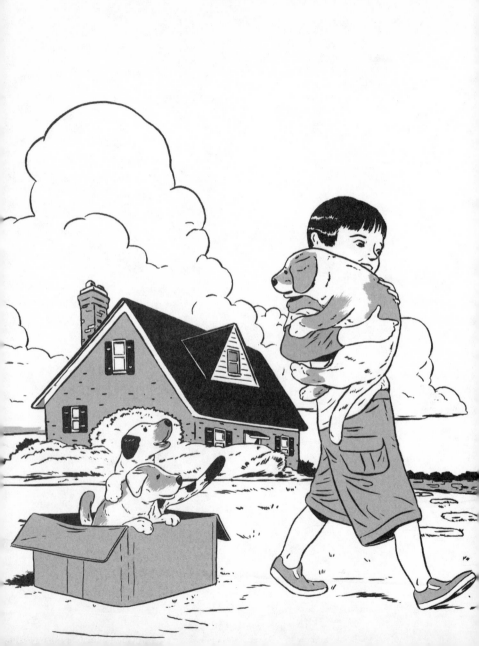

# Extreme Youth

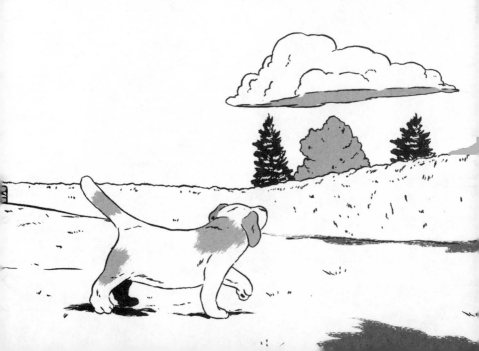

# Mortification
# at the Fall Fair

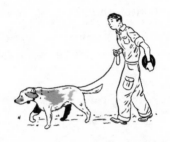

I went to *Best of Show* by accident. We were told to go to
some other movie by one of the kids—"You *have* to see
it!"—and so, like obedient parents, we shuffled off to the
local cinema with its twenty-four screens and ten-deep
lineups. Perhaps the line went on too long. Whatever—
when I finally got to the window I'd forgotten the title
we just *had* to see and said, "Two for *Best of Show*, please."

It was a happy screw-up. *Best of Show* is about a New York
dog competition, a movie about eccentric breeders and
posh kennel clubs and strange-looking animals and

their equally strange-looking handlers. It is fiction but intended to feel like a documentary—and it is hilarious. Fred Willard plays a colour analyst called "Buck" Laughlin, and when he isn't going on about his proctologist he's making the most wildly inappropriate comments, such as, "I went to one of those obedience places once—*it was all going well until they spilled hot candle wax on my private parts!*"

But it wasn't anything Buck said that sent me spinning back in time. It was a very quick, somewhat funny comment by another actor, whose dog suddenly reaches up to lick his face during the competition. *"Don't!"* he shouts out. *"Not the lips!"*

Sitting there watching *Best of Show,* I drifted back to my own singular experience with a dog show. I would say what year it was, but readers might then wonder how I could possibly still be alive. So please just accept that it was a long time ago and involved Cindy, a dog no longer with us—so she cannot be embarrassed by this story. And mercifully, there was no Buck Laughlin around at the Huntsville Fall Fair to offer running commentary on the incident.

I had a new puppy at a time when it seemed as if there wasn't a kid along Reservoir Hill who didn't come with a dog. Cindy was a cute little thing with blond, curling fur. She was close to a spaniel, but without the bobbed tail. Brent and Ron next door had Buster, who had what appeared to be a healthy mix of hound, husky, shepherd and, given its small size, perhaps dachshund. Donnie up the street had Ric, so close to a German shepherd that it might even have been a purebred—surely the only one in town—but I don't ever remember anyone mentioning papers or anything. Sinclair, across Mary Street from Brent and Ron, had Lady, a bright little poodle-terrier mix and considerably older than the other dogs. Bob, down Mary Street a bit, had Queenie, a sister of Buster.

There was a notice on the telephone pole that stood at the corner of Lorne and Mary streets between Bob's house and Brent's.

*Huntsville Fall Fair Dog Show!*
*Children Under 12 Only! Cash Prizes!*

We read it and could not believe it. The annual fair was coming to town—midways, animals, sideshows, candy floss, thrill rides—and the chance to get into the fair for free and maybe even win a little money for the midway was irresistible. We all decided to enter. Each one of us who owned a dog.

It is difficult in a time of twenty-four-screen theatres to describe just what the fall fair coming to a small town once meant. It was a day off for the schools. The students lined up, class by class, and marched the entire length of Main Street, up Brunel Road and down past the hockey rink to the fairgrounds. The high school marching band led the parade, the mayor rode in a convertible, and there were floats for everything from the 4-H Club to the contestants who would be competing to be named Fall Fair Princess.

It was a time for stretching imaginations, for suspending disbelief, for opening up any and all possibilities, from the chance of getting the cute girl up the street onto the merry-go-round to running away with the midway.

Those of us who made up what was known as the Mary Street Gang had once stood in line to pay our quarters—a considerable sum in those days for ten- and eleven-year-olds—for the opportunity to enter a pitch-black tent and stare, hopelessly, into a dark pool that held "The Hippo That Sweats Blood!" We could hear something sloshing around in the dark, but had not the slightest proof that it was a hippopotamus. It had to be, though. The man outside said it was. And we had paid good money for the right to see one of the greatest mysteries of the world.

The hippo, the man said, had to be kept constantly in a pool of oil. If we listened, we could hear him moving about. We listened; we heard something. We took the man at his word. "We cannot reveal this strange and unusual creature to the sunlight!" he shouted in the darkness. "He has to be kept in the dark. He has to live in dark oil, not water. If the sun shines on him, he will sweat. And if he sweats, he *dies*—cruelly drained of his life juices!"

Well, who could argue with that? Did any of us want a dead hippo—especially the only one in the world that sweats blood—on his conscience? Of course not. We simply filed out, not questioning the man, and promptly headed off to tell others that we had seen one of the great wonders of the world.

You never knew what would happen at a Huntsville Fall Fair. Sometimes there were stories you wanted to tell, like "The Hippo That Sweats Blood," and sometimes there were stories you prayed no one would ever tell. Like the Day of the Dog Show.

THAT DAY we all gathered at Brent and Ron's with our dogs. Mine was, by far, the youngest of the assembled dogs, a puppy still in the early stages of training. But Cindy was so friendly she fit in, even with the bigger and much older dogs like Ric, the shepherd. We had no idea what to expect. The notice nailed up on the telephone pole had said nothing about specifics. Just "Dog Show," and that was good enough for us. We figured it would have to do with walking the dogs back and forth, making them sit and perhaps even stay. Donnie advised, and we all agreed, that we should carry small dog biscuits in our pockets as rewards for the dogs. It seemed a sensible thing to do. So we filled our pockets from a bag in Brent and Ron's kitchen and set out for the fairgrounds and arena.

We knew the arena well. It was where we played hockey in winter and lacrosse in summer. A few of us from Reservoir Hill even had our team pictures up on the walls. It was a place of great memories—up until the dog show.

They had us assemble with our dogs behind the stands, waiting to be called out. We were practically the only entries, the five dogs of Reservoir Hill and two other dogs, one handled by a young girl in a church dress, from another part of town. We barely knew the other kids entering. We said nothing to them and they said nothing to us. Our dogs snarled at theirs and their dogs barked at ours. Neighbourhoods were like that in those days.

They held the preliminaries for the Fall Fair Princess and then announced the dog show. The man announcing— a large, pot-bellied man also, unfortunately, named

Roy—wore dark pants and red suspenders over a white shirt, his sleeves rolled up and held by black barber's bands, with a small dark fedora, looking as if it had been punched, set far back on his head. His teeth were as yellowed, chipped, and crooked as the tombstones at the pioneer cemetery. He showed them a lot because, even before the dog show began, he seemed to think it was funny.

They gave us numbers. Donnie was first, with Ric. I was last, seventh, with Cindy. It was fortunate that they gave Donnie and Ric number one. Donnie was the best of us all with dogs; Ric was the smartest. The man called Roy brought Donnie out and had him walk Ric about the stage. Big and dark and elegant, Ric moved about gracefully, the leash looping to show it was not even necessary, and appreciative applause went up from the crowd.

Some of us peeked around from behind the tarpaulin screen that stood between the stage and the staging area for the dogs and their owners. I could see faces in the crowd that I knew. There were more people there than I had expected—What else was there to do on a fall evening in a small town that got only one television channel and had but a single theatre?—and I shuddered, suddenly wishing I could be anywhere else but here at that precise moment with my excitable little untrained puppy.

The Master of Ceremonies then had Donnie do some basic tricks with Ric. He had Donnie make Ric sit, which Ric did perfectly. Then shake a paw. Perfect again, and Donnie slipped Ric one of his dog biscuits.

"Show us how your dog will stay," Roy instructed.

Donnie nodded. He had Ric sit first. He pointed forcefully at him. *"Stay!"* he commanded. Ric stayed. Donnie walked completely across the stage, his back to the dog, and then turned. Ric stayed.

"How about *that?!*" the man called Roy barked into his microphone. The arena exploded in applause and cheers. You would think Donnie—or perhaps Ric—had just scored in overtime.

Donnie and Ric left to applause, and the MC began working through the numbers. Brent and Ron argued about who should go out with Buster, and eventually Brent did and Buster did a fair loop of the stage and not much more. But since the man called Roy seemed to know Brent, or more likely Brent and Ron's popular father, Maurice, an appliance salesman at the local Eaton's store, he congratulated Brent on his fine-looking dog and the crowd seemed to agree.

The boy from another part of town went out and his dog performed fairly well, though kept barking. Sinc went out with Lady, and Lady, one of the smartest dogs I have ever known, was virtually flawless, almost as if she'd studied Ric and was doing exactly as she'd seen the big shepherd do.

They called out number five, Bob and his dog Queenie, and Queenie froze at the tarp and refused to go out at all. Bob yanked on his leash, but the dog, a powerful little mutt with wide shoulders, put down her haunches and absolutely refused. Bob pulled, Queenie refused, the man called Roy called them out again. The crowd laughed. And finally Bob leaned around the tarp and said that his dog refused to come.

"Okay, then," the man called Roy boomed into the microphone, "we have a disqualification. Dog says it doesn't 'do it' in front of crowds." The crowd howled with laughter. Bob begged and pulled; Queenie still held fast. I could not imagine a worse situation.

The other strange kid, the girl, now went out and her little dog also balked. But since it was so much smaller and less powerful than Queenie she was able to get it out onto the stage, where the crowd laughed and cheered. She then dragged—*dragged*—the poor little thing from one side of the stage to the other.

"Well," said the man called Roy, "that dog certainly goes where you tell it to, don't it?" The crowd roared. All the others, Bob included, were laughing at the poor girl with the dog, her cheeks beet red with embarrassment. She tried to make the dog stay, and this time it did move with her when she walked away. The crowd roared with laughter again. It can't possibly get worse than this, I thought. It could, and did.

Finally the girl with the reluctant dog came back through the curtain formed by the tarpaulin, the crowd cheering her as she left. She seemed to me to be near tears.

"And now for our final contestant of the night," the man called Roy barked into the microphone. "Roy—good name, that!—and his Wonder Dog, Cindy!"

I pulled and Cindy balked. I'd expected that. She was shy and still just a puppy. I tugged again and this time Cindy came with me.

We rounded the tarpaulin and came out onto the stage. It was, to me, a shock. The lights, the warmth, the sea of smiling faces, the huge powerful presence of the man called Roy and his microphone, the sense that Cindy and I were trapped.

"Walk her around now," the man called Roy ordered. I did, and Cindy came fairly well. A warm round of applause rippled through the crowd.

"Let's see if she'll stay," the man called Roy said. I tried to do as Donnie had done to Ric. I stood and pointed firmly at her.

"Stay!" I commanded. I backed away. Cindy came with me. I remembered the biscuits, pulled one out, and dropped it. Some in the crowd laughed. I picked it up and tried again. *"Stay!"* I yelled. I must have frightened her, because when I backed away she jumped from her haunches and then dipped back down again.

Something fell from her rear end. I realized immediately what it was. It was as if my face had been dipped in a boiling kettle.

The man called Roy noticed, too. "Well," he barked into the microphone. "What do we have here? Is that another 'dog biscuit' on the stage, Roy?"

The crowd roared.

I had no idea what to say. I backed farther away, Cindy followed, but first dipping again and dropping something else on the stage.

"Biscuits are coming fast and furious here!" the man called Roy announced to another roar of the crowd. Cindy still had another in her. "And another!" he announced, giving a play-by-play of her lack of toilet training.

I was mortified. I grabbed her leash and we scrambled off the stage to more roars and laughter.

The man called Roy was still talking. "We'll have the presentation, ladies and gentlemen, soon's we get these ... dog biscuits ... cleaned off the stage here!"

I had played dozens of hockey games and lacrosse games in this same arena, but never heard such cheering as followed the man called Roy's endless witticisms about the "biscuits" that had fallen from poor Cindy. I wanted to leave right away but my friends, who were also laughing at me, were all staying. I wanted to cry, but they were all looking, and I couldn't possibly.

I leaned down and picked up Cindy. I hugged her hard. She was shaking like a leaf.

The man called Roy was calling out the judges' decisions. "First place, seven dollars, goes to Donnie and his dog Ric." Donnie and Ric bounded back out onto the stage. "Second place and six dollars goes to Sinclair and his dog Lady." Off went Sinc and Lady to collect their booty.

I burned even more with envy. Seven bucks, or six bucks, would pay for an entire day on the midway. Rides, candy, games—perhaps they'd even win something at one of those games where you tried to land a ping-pong ball in a small goldfish bowl or something.

Down through the line they went. Brent and Ron won. The other kids won.

"Sixth place, and two dollars, goes to our biscuit boy, Roy and Cindy!" I heard my name, heard the laughter, and found I was being pushed out onto the stage, Cindy staying behind with Brent while I collected. "Careful where you step now!" the man called Roy commanded. He pretended to jump away from something. "*Hey*—that a fresh *biscuit* or a fresh something else?"

The crowd howled once more. I grabbed my two-dollar bill—this was when there was still such a thing in this country—and virtually ran off stage.

"And last place, one dollar," the man called Roy announced, "goes to Bob and the little dog that wouldn't come out, Queenie." Laughing, Bob bounded out onto the stage, grabbed his money, and hurried back. We were all winners. Sort of.

Soon it didn't matter at all. We all had our money. Ric and Lady were the stars. And no one was saying anything cruel about Cindy, who after all was no more than a puppy. The five of us and our five dogs walked home together, up past the high school, up the street and onto Reservoir Hill.

I got home and showed my mother the two-dollar bill that Cindy and I had won at the fall fair dog show, but I never said a word about the biscuits incident and the way the crowd had laughed at us.

"You better get to bed," she said. "It's late."

It was, now well past ten. I called Cindy and let her out once more before the night—though after her performance on the public stage, it hardly seemed necessary—and then let her back in and leaned down to pat her and hug her before she curled up on the old blanket in the back room. I wondered if she had any realization, or memory, of what had happened. I wondered if a dog, like a cat, can be embarrassed. I wondered what she thought of the horrible thing I had just put her through.

But she was no different this night from any other night at bedtime. She took the pats on the head and the scratches of the ears and moaned and wiggled and, suddenly, put her front paws on my crouching knees and leaned up, tail wagging, and licked me.

Right on the lips.

# Shoes
# and Socks

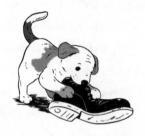

Choices, choices, choices. The garbage needs putting out, so I could put on a right roller skate and a left running shoe. Or a left slipper and a right winter boot.

Soon I have to go out myself, which means tracking down a right and a left dress shoe and hoping they're the same colour. Fortunately, there are only two pairs, one black and one brown, so the chances of matching colours—presuming I can find a right and a left—are somewhat improved. Later on I have hockey, and mercifully the skates are inside their own zippered pouches—

but even so, I'd better check. Just to make sure I don't end up stepping on the ice with one left skate and one right snowshoe.

It was never this way before the puppy arrived.

All dogs have nervous disorders. Some immediately fall over and turn up their stomach. Some hump your leg. Some pee when they meet strangers. Some even lunge for the throat. This one called Willow, five months old and looking like no breed ever before known to man or dogkind, has to have a shoe in her mouth. It is the oddest thing. The slightest excitement—a knock at the door, a kid arriving home from work, a loud commercial—and the puppy will suddenly appear, wildly wiggling, with a shoe in her mouth. It may be the last time you see the shoe, or its match, for days.

None of this makes the slightest sense. She does not chew the shoes, but merely holds them in her mouth until, at some point of neurotic comfort, she decides to stop her wiggling and drop the shoe somewhere, anywhere, and move on.

And it is not as if a shoe is all there is around here to serve as a pacifier. Because there are no longer very young children around, and because there are now almost as many pet stores in the country as there are Tim Hortons, she has an endless supply of toys to turn to in stressful moments. There are ducks and penguins that squeak, furry rabbits that honk, footballs, red-white-and-blue balls, Frisbees, plastic bones, rope pulls, and fake squirrels. There is even a rubber shoe—which, incidentally, holds not the slightest interest for her.

The vanishing shoes have brought back memories of that brilliant, long-ago episode of *Married With Children* in which Al Bundy becomes convinced that his socks are going missing because green aliens are sneaking into the Bundy home at night and taking them to use as fuel for their spaceships.

"Peg!" Al shouts at one point. "Three little aliens came in here and ... they stole my socks!"

"Were they green before or after they touched your socks?" Peg asks.

Al, much to the shock of Peg, turns out to be right. The aliens were, in fact, green and were, indeed, after mizzoozzoo—alien talk for "fuel." Al's stinky socks proved to be exactly what was required to send ships off to intercept a giant comet hurtling straight for Earth—which made for another happy ending for *Married With Children*.

Poor Al might have been laughed at here on Earth, but, according to a trailer that followed the program, "On planet Philydion, they still sing songs of the man who made it possible for the comet to be destroyed. The man who saved Earth and a hundred worlds by providing fuel for the ships which diverted the comet. And that man is … Al Bundy." Brings a tear to the eye, doesn't it?

There are, however, no little green men around here, just a young mutt that steals the cats' food for *mizzoozzoo* and isn't comfortable unless someone's shoe is hanging from her mouth.

The search for missing shoes has, naturally, brought up the third most perplexing puzzle humans have been known to ponder since the beginning of time. The first, obviously, is "Who created God?" (For the answer, please turn to page 368.) The second, and more recent puzzle, is "If people truly get the politicians they deserve, what did we do to deserve this?" And the third, of course, is the Mystery of the Lone Shoe.

The Lone Shoe is a conundrum considered by everyone who has ever driven a car on a busy freeway and wondered why there is only one sneaker in the fast lane. It is a question debated internally by everyone who has ever looked into a ditch and wondered how such a fine-looking sandal, single, came to be lying there.

There are, in any given community at any given moment, more single, lonely shoes than Imelda Marcos has pairs. There are, around this world, entire monuments erected to the Mystery of the Lone Shoe, single sneakers and sandals and baby shoes and rubber boots hanging by their laces as if, absurdly, expecting a mate to show up unexpectedly. There are websites featuring the Mystery of the Lone Shoe. People in chat rooms trade theories on their existence. There are even eccentrics who go around photographing lone shoes at roadsides.

One successful writer, David Feldman, a man obsessed with unanswerable questions (which he calls "frustables"), has apparently devoted seven pages of his book *When Do Fish Sleep?* to the Lone Shoe phenomenon. I have not seen the book and now do not need to, for the answer is, at this very moment, curled up on a small mat at my feet, sleeping beside a lone shoe.

The answer is, obviously, neurotic puppies—the lone shoe fetish perhaps the only genetic stream that is traceable in this curious creature that looks far more like a fox than the border collie the owner of its mother predicted. Crazy, insecure puppies everywhere, each with a single shoe in the mouth every time the doorbell rings. The other shoe is off travelling somewhere on its own, perhaps never to be seen again.

# The
# Puppy Brain

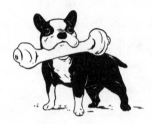

Come join us on a tour of the puppy brain. It's a walking tour, so watch where you step, please.

My own experience, garnered from years of reporting on Parliament Hill, is to deal with brains that spend every waking minute thinking of ways to stay in, or get back in—so it is quite something to consider a brain, of roughly equal size, that spends every waking minute thinking of how to get *out*.

We will begin the tour by entering through the ear. Again, careful as you step. Beware that slashing back paw.

And pay no attention to that odd-looking bug hiding in the hair below where the paw is raking—it's just about to go off and lay some eggs in the living room rug anyway. You will note that the ears of this particular model, known around here as "Bandit," make no sense. The size would seem to come from Labrador, the flop from border collie, the colour from Dalmatian, and the cocky twist of the left ear probably from that male terrier who broke loose down along the Ottawa River last March. He's the one they say is responsible for all this in the first place.

Those receivers you see set up all around the ear channel are extremely sophisticated, so try not to touch, if you don't mind. They are highly sensitive and capable of hearing a mailman at two hundred paces, a hand being formed into a fist for knocking at the front door, a squirrel leaping from branch to branch half a block away—but they cannot, for some reason, ever seem to pick up the sound of its own name, no matter how loudly shouted or, indeed, screamed.

Directly through the ear is a short tunnel leading to open sky. That odd swooshing sound you hear—a bit like gusting wind—is the commands and orders and calls and, well, out-and-out begging from me going in one ear and out the other.

Here, just to the side, we will find the seven-month-old puppy's sensory centre. So far, it understands but one word: "walk." It is a word that these sensory organs can pick up at fifty paces even if whispered, even if attached to another word, like "sidewalk," even if intended as nothing more than an innocent discussion of the apparatus required to cook vegetables Chinese style. Alarms have been known to go off even if the word is spelled out: "w ... a ... l ... k." Science has no explanation.

Next door to the sensory centre we come to the small package of cells that control motor movement and go into action the moment the leash is attached to the collar. Once these cells swing into action, the front legs are instructed never to touch the ground, the throat is directed to issue only death rattles, and the nose is commanded to lead the desperate lunge for all the latest toilet gossip of the neighbourhood.

The puppy view of reality is contained in a single, twisted cell—very tiny, you'll see it hiding in that crevice over there—that believes all humans secretly desire to have forty-pound dogs jumping at their faces, are highly impressed by barking, and like nothing better than to see a dog giving its private parts a good and thorough licking.

Over there to the left is the taste centre of the puppy brain. That blackboard on the wall listing today's specials includes a morning round of used Kleenex, a teenager's sock that should have been washed a week ago, a Barbie doll head, the inside of a perfectly good slipper, cat food, three chicken bones from the garbage, a slice of processed cheese—still wrapped in plastic—that someone was dumb enough to leave on the table, a bowlful of Lite-Brite markers, several ankles, the mail, one library book, and a beer conveniently knocked over by a wagging tail.

One floor above taste, we come to the room that contains all the ambitions of a seven-month-old puppy brain. In ascending order, the room contains (i) a hope that the garage door is open to the garbage, (ii) that the big German shepherd by the bike path gets run over, (iii) that they get tired of booting me off the chesterfield and, above all, (iv) a growing hope that now that they've stopped putting me off the bed I'll get my own pillow.

There is, just off a bit to the right, a very tiny mass of cells that contains the puppy logic. It is, at seven months, fully developed. It believes that one solves the problem of a chain wrapping around a tree by continuing in precisely the same direction until it is wrapped four times and there is barely enough slack left to permit howling. It also believes, in this instance, that, like the two cats in this house, it, too, fits perfectly on any size lap.

Finally, we should spend some time puzzling over one of the great mysteries of the universe: the puppy view of sex. Two months ago, there was no view. Then one day a nice car ride turned into a guy in a white jacket with a needle, total darkness, and then waking up with stitches to lick. Since that moment, the legs of passing strangers have taken on a new and highly attractive appearance. Visitors are therefore once again advised to watch their step as they leave. For what they might land in—as well as what might land on them.

# Care and Feeding, Then and Now

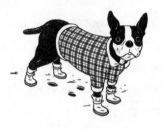

I have been in love with dogs ever since I stumbled on a litter of black puppies in a back shed at Aunt Minnie's many, many years ago. Aunt Minnie, actually Great Aunt Minnie, lived on a small farm deep in the Ottawa Valley. She had a well rather than running water and coal oil lamps rather than electricity, but she also had a place of fabulous wealth in the eyes of a young child: chickens and roosters in the yard, cows in the back fields, once in a while a pig, and cats and dogs everywhere—but not in the house. That is how it was then. Dogs lived outside; or, if they were lucky, in a shed.

Aunt Minnie had lived a long and healthy life and was around ninety when she died at her little farm. They held the funeral there, too, Aunt Minnie laid out in a casket in the sitting room, keeners moaning on chairs along the far wall, the women sitting in the dining room tinkling spoons against their tea cups, and the men gathered in the woodshed tinkling their tonsils with cheap whisky straight from the bottle.

A child not comfortable in either group, and most assuredly not comfortable with the casket and the keeners in the sitting room, fled naturally to the outside. Being the only kid at the funeral—taken simply because I was too small to be left with neighbours, as my older brother and sister had been—I had headed out into the barnyard to be, as a far superior writer once put it, "young and easy under the apple boughs / About the lilting house and happy as the grass was green."

Aunt Minnie's farm had a half dozen sheds. Some held chickens, some held old machinery, some held hay, some manure, some milk cans and bottles, some nothing but flaking swallows' nests and active beehives. One, however, held the preserves she put down each summer—wild raspberry and blueberry jams, pickled cucumbers and beans and carrots and onions—and there, in the middle of the floor, was half a wooden crate filled with the most magical toys I have ever come across.

Six black puppies.

The mother, whose name I forget but not the look, was a mutt with black curling hair and floppy ears. She must have had a touch of spaniel, a bit of collie. She was gentle and friendly and lived her life out and about the barnyard, though had been allowed inside the shed attached to the house to care for her litter.

The puppies were still nursing. They must have been three or four weeks old, for they tumbled and jumped with their paws and needle-sharp teeth at a small boy's lap as he knelt and played with them for so long his mother had to leave the tea group and come and find him so he'd be cleaned up for the funeral and the long walk—Aunt Minnie's sons and sons-in-law and nephews carrying the casket—down to the little church on the shore of the Bonnechere River.

The puppies mesmerized me. I remember begging my mother to let me take one, but one of the men who overheard us said the puppies weren't yet weaned—whatever that meant—and we'd have to wait a couple of weeks before they could be taken from their mother. I asked if we could get one then and my mother answered as she usually did when the ultimate answer was bound to be no: "We'll see."

We didn't see because we didn't get back to Aunt Minnie's that summer. It wasn't many summers after that, however, that another litter showed up closer to home and "We'll see" became, as it usually did after enough begging and whining and pleading and even crying, "Okay."

"Okay, but you'll have to take care of it yourself."

"Of course," I answered, insulted that such a statement would even be necessary.

It was necessary, of course, and perhaps she should have had a written legal contract as well, because as all parents eventually discover, the raising of their children's pets usually falls, at some point, to them.

It is hard to believe how much the care of animals has changed since then—even for those of us who neglected our promises. The dogs of Aunt Minnie's litter never saw the inside of a house. The dogs of my first litter did, but only in back rooms or basements. Dogs were then trained by discipline—a rolled-up newspaper for punishment; a snout placed in, or almost in, an accident to make sure it didn't happen again, though it usually did; a choke chain to teach them to heel. I had a friend named Fred who trained his nippy puppy not to bite by picking the thing up in both his hands and sinking his own choppers into the puppy's neck until it yelped so loud it seemed Fred had bitten it in half.

Those dogs learned not to bite, learned to go outside to pee, learned not to wreck furniture or tear apart shoes—but they would never be taught that way today.

My first dog was kept in a basement, a dirt-floor basement with a bare bulb hanging down off the ceiling for light, much of the basement jammed thick with slabwood from the local mill that we burned in a furnace. My second dog was kept outside in a doghouse in summer and in a back room in winter. My third and fourth dogs had the run of the house and slept where they wished. My fifth prefers to be crated at night.

My first dog had a leash and collar from Stedman's five-and-dime store, both cheap. My fifth dog has a variety of leashes and a couple of stylish collars from a suburban box store for pets. A daughter's dog—in many ways my sixth, it seems—has a variety of clothes, including faux fur by "Fursacci" and little booties for when she heads outside in winter. Come Christmas, she has a complete Santa's outfit to wear for the occasion.

My first dog, Buddy, was fed scraps. My second dog, Cindy, a combination of scraps and this new "kibble" that was on the market. My third, Bumps, and fourth, Bandit, had kibble and, for special moments, canned dog food. My fifth, Willow, just came begging for a treat, which I fetched for her and for my daughter's little Boston terrier, Cricket.

Salmon Sushi Dog Treats. I plead insanity.

# Fetch...
## Fetch... Fetch...

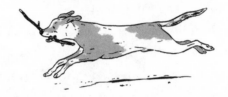

I know only his first name, Matt, but I need to find him.
My lawyer wants to serve him.

The end of my life as I know it came a week ago when
this young man named Matt did nothing more than pick
up a stick and throw it. It didn't hit me, but there are
times when I wish it had—like at 3:42 yesterday morning
when, without warning, a bundle of thick white and
brown fur came flying through the bedroom doorway
and landed full force on my chest and stayed there. It
being approximately the surface temperature of Venus

(480°C) outside and there being no air conditioning, a fur blanket was about the last thing I was interested in. It was, however, somewhat less annoying than hearing, and feeling, the unmistakable plop of a tennis ball as it hit my shoulder and rolled, with uncanny accuracy, down toward my throwing hand.

Perhaps I should describe this tennis ball so that you can appreciate the full impact of what it felt like. It is the third tennis ball to be pulled from the new package from the dollar store in the past two days. It began life, as all the tennis balls have, clean and green and soft. Within a matter of minutes, however, it became, like all those before it, black and wet and slimy, great gobs of goo and sand and dirt and heaven knows what else hanging from it as it rides about in the mouth of this eight-month-old puppy named Willow.

The ball, incidentally, has just landed on my keyboard, so excuse me for a bit while I get the Windex and paper towels and then go outside for an hour or two of wrecking the rotator cuff.

I do not know what it is that Matt unleashed when he picked up that first stick and threw it. It's hardly as if the dog had never fetched anything before—though it must be admitted that she rarely brought anything back—but it was as if her age and his stick-throwing suddenly came together the way VLTs and hard liquor sometimes do for humans. Willow was hooked.

The big difference is that if someone else suddenly becomes transfixed with VLTs, it is not necessary for me to go along and push the flashing buttons that start the cherries spinning. Not so with fetching. If the dog gets hooked, the owner becomes an unwilling addict.

I have tried to figure out how this happened. We were at the lake. We were visiting friends on the other side of the island. The barbecue was on. The beer was ice cold. Matt, the nephew of our friends, seemed to be a nice, friendly, sensible young man right up until the moment he reached down, picked up a piece of broken branch, and hurled it off into the woods. The dog chased it down, brought it back, Matt threw it once again, and the rest is history.

Hooked. Addicted. Totally obsessed as I have never before seen a dog become. (There is another dog around our summer place this year, a daughter's Boston terrier, but its only obsession is passing wind that would fell a hemlock.)

The puppy is a mutt. No one, not even its mother's owner, can figure out its lineage. She has the one blue eye of an Australian sheepdog, but the crouching, heel-nipping, and herding instincts of a border collie. This is fine with me. In the past, I have been more than happy to have one around to round up little swimmers who dare venture beyond the drop-off. None of the others, however, had to have something in the mouth. Always. Every waking moment.

First it was shoes, but now, even if you pop up at dawn, she is at the door with a stick or tennis ball being lolled about the mouth as though it were some precious jewel no one could resist reaching for. She is ready to fetch at midnight, ready—as I discovered several hours back—to fetch at 3:42 A.M.

I have tried various solutions. Someone in the house

went to one of those new pet megastores—you know, the ones that make the West Edmonton Mall look like a corner store—and returned with a plastic "arm" that you load and that fires the ball with greater ease than a real arm. And at one point I even got out my old lacrosse stick and began tossing the ball so far into the bush that it seemed not even embedded GPS and satellite tracking would find it, all to no avail. In a moment Willow was back, black tongue dragging on the ground, sides frantically panting, ball in mouth so black and goopered there was no longer a hint of green to be seen.

I turned to the internet. On one site, a veterinarian talking about obsessive-compulsive behaviour offers the line, "Women think men have a one-track mind ... that is, until they meet a border collie." Another professional, a dog psychologist it seems, operating out of New York City, suggests Prozac as a possible cure. For the puppy or the owner? The site isn't clear. Either way, a frightening thought.

But not quite so alarming, perhaps, as the soggy black ball that has once again been plunked in my lap. And even if there were such a pill around here, and it was meant for the pet not the human, there is still one problem. How, I wonder, would you ever get it past a mouth that is plugged twenty-four hours a day with a tennis ball?

# The
# Teen Years

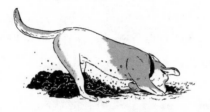

Seven for every one. The rule of thumb—rule of dewclaw, if you prefer—for measuring dog years against human years is to count seven human years for every one dog year. There is a point, admittedly, where this works fairly well. A nine-year-old mutt, for example, is much the same as a sixty-three-year-old human mongrel. A fifteen-year-old pooch is very much a centenarian with teeth and bladder problems. It falls apart, however, when trying to figure out puppies.

The current subject—the one sleeping in the corner over there with all four paws in the air—will be closing in on a year some time before Christmas. The date is inexact, as might be expected of a mutt of uncertain lineage that a mischievous daughter found in a distant Humane Society. But if we guess ten or eleven months, then this creature named Willow, by the accepted measure, should be roughly kinder-garten level.

I don't think so. For one thing, she is too stupid. For another thing, she is too smart.

The seven-for-one math simply does not work in the first year of a dog's life. What human, for example, can walk at two weeks? What human can chew, and partly digest, a shoe at four weeks? What human has ever been known to run away at eight weeks? Find me the human baby who can swim across a bay at six months, let alone a beginning toddler who can chase a car halfway to work at ten months. Show me the child, please, who is house-trained at seven months—well, partly house-trained, anyway.

Then again, we do not—at least I hope not—see a six-month-old baby insisting on hanging about the house with a dirty sock in her mouth. We do not find an infant demanding cat food instead of the food intended for her. We do not see toddlers taking apart, stitch by stitch, every toy they are ever shown to chomp down and burst the plastic squeaker inside.

It is a difficult measure, admittedly, but I think there is a simple solution: triple the rule of thumb for the first year and, if the dog reaches fifteen, forget even trying and just start treating every extra year as an extra year. By this methodology, it is safe to conclude that the brown and white creature sighing in the corner is a ... teenager. Certainly, the signs are irrefutable:

- Gets up, eats, goes back to sleep, gets up, goes out, comes in, eats, sleeps, whines if can't go out in evening, eats, sleeps.
- Never picks up after herself. There are mismatched socks everywhere, including one in her mouth.

There are chewed balls, destroyed squeaky toys, pull toys, animal toys strewn everywhere. If you place them neatly back in her toy box, she spends fifteen minutes hauling them out and placing them, randomly, where they are most likely to be in the way.

· Totally, one hundred percent self-absorbed. It is all "me ... me ... *ME!*" all the time. She wants fed, wants out, wants in, wants petted, wants someone to play with her, wants on the bed, wants on the furniture, wants in the refrigerator, wants the cats' food, wants the humans' food, wants to roll in whatever she can find—dead squirrel, crushed groundhog, rotted bird carcass....

· Single-minded. If you have seen a teenage human hypnotized, transfixed, and obsessed with a video game, you will have some sense—some very small sense—of what it's like to see a dog willing to chase a ball or stick much longer than the human arm can throw.

· Megalomania. What does it tell you when a dog stops and looks around the field if she happens to catch a thrown ball on the first bounce? What does it tell you when a dog insists on walking through the woods with a log big enough to take down a hiker at the back of the knees? Or when the dog insists on bounding past you just as the trail becomes wide enough for one? What does it say to you when a skinny little puppy suddenly tries to puff up like an Arctic sled dog the moment any other dog comes along the trail?

· Whining. Whine to get out, whine to get in. Whine to be fed, whine for more. Whine for a treat, whine for a second treat. Whine to get out, whine to get in. Whine to play, whine to play, whine to play, whine to play....

· Stubborn. Approximately once a week does as she is told. Other 4,587 times it's a toss-up. Shall I "come" or shall I scoot? Shall I "sit" or shall I lunge? As for "stay"—don't even think about it.

· Driving. Insists on sitting in best seat. Would prefer driver's seat if available. Wants windows down so she can hang head out.

· Clumsy. Fine to hang your head out the car window, but not so fine, she will surely eventually realize, to place paw on automatic window and set reverse guillotine in motion....

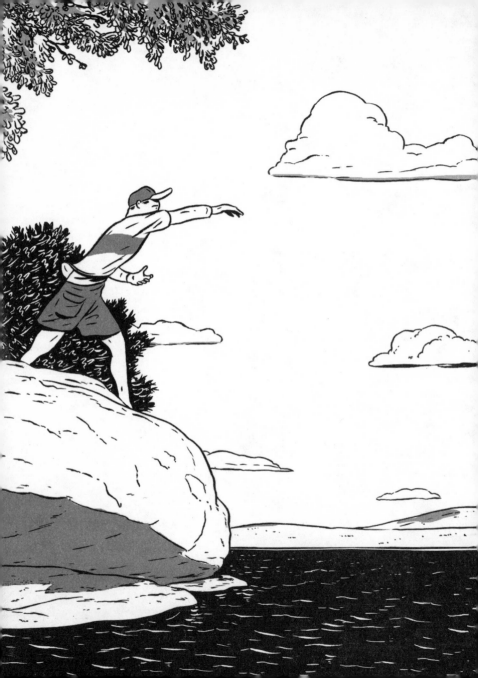

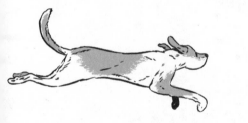

# Alleged Adulthood

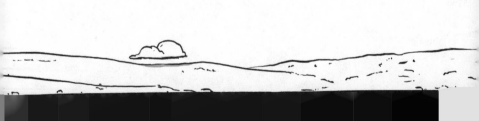

# Pawprinted Legacies
# of the Great

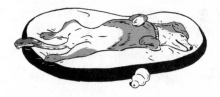

I have started reading to my dog. Not stuff I have written—
there is, after all, a Humane Society in this town—but
self-improvement books. *Her* self-improvement.

And why not read? Everyone talks to the dog. I even
saw a poll somewhere that claimed one out of every three
of us telephones the dog—homesick travellers calling
back to have whoever answers hold out the receiver while
the deranged traveller tries to coax a bark out of the
poor dumbfounded thing. Reading, however, has a far
more honourable purpose than the self-gratification of

a business traveller feeling sorry for himself. I want this dog—this one-year-old mutt called Willow, who is just beginning to come into her own—to become something special, not just something I call home to talk to when nobody else will listen.

The dog needs inspiration. It lay, asleep, legs in the air, the other morning while one of the many unemployed in this house watched *The Ellen DeGeneres Show*. A man was on talking about how, out walking one evening with his Labradors, he had fallen into a diabetic coma. The yellow Lab lay on him to keep the man warm while the black Lab—I'm not making this up; I'm not allowed to—grabbed the flashlight the man had dropped and began running about the field with it in its mouth until a policeman noticed the dancing light and came to investigate.

Thanks to the dogs, the policeman's CPR, and an ambulance, the man's life was saved. When he came back from hospital, he told Ellen, the dogs began to weep.

This dog sleeping on the floor, on the other hand, would pick up a flashlight only if someone first threw it.

And then she'd want it thrown again and again and again and again until, frankly, the thrower might welcome a diabetic coma.

Perhaps it's the breed. A couple of months ago, while travelling in the United States, I came across an advice column for pet owners. A woman had written in to say her new dog's constant staring had "weirded" her out to the point where she'd decided to take the little border collie back to the kennel where she got it. The advice columnist, bless his heart, gloriously ripped into her, saying the breed is *supposed* to stare like that. Such dogs, the expert said, are extremely bright. It wasn't staring but rather looking for a signal to do something—like fetch, or round up the sheep—and the only thing dumb about border collies is that they think humans have enough intelligence to offer direction.

This dog isn't quite a border collie, but she is enough of one to stare endlessly in search of a stick or ball that might fly through the air and have to be instantly returned for the next throw. And the next. And the next ...

So, being a fairly bright human compared with the woman who took her dog back, I have decided to take that columnist's sage advice and offer direction. Which is why I have started reading to my dog. The book we have chosen is *The Pawprints of History* by Stanley Coren, a professor of psychology at the University of British Columbia. Subtitled *Dogs and the Course of Human Events,* the book was a gift from a friend—and we are most grateful for its inspiration.

I have explained to Willow that I expect great things from her, but I am not expecting the impossible. It would be unlikely, for example, that she might ever start her own church, though Stanley Coren makes an excellent case that the very existence of Protestantism is directly tied to the intervention of a greyhound called Urian.

According to the Coren interpretation of religious history, Protestantism would never have been necessary to invent had Pope Clement VII only seen fit to grant Henry VIII the divorce he was seeking in order to marry the charming Anne Boleyn. All that was required was for the Pope to grant an annulment on whatever cocked-up and cooked-up basis would suffice. The king dispatched his main churchman, Cardinal Thomas Wolsey, off to Rome to ask the favour and Wolsey, a great dog lover, insisted on taking along Urian, his rather overprotective pet.

Custom demanded that supplicants approach the papal throne and kiss the Pope's toe. Wolsey, a good Catholic and a Cardinal, naturally had no difficulty with this, but poor Urian misunderstood the bare foot swinging out toward his master's lips, leapt over his master, and smartly bit Pope Clement VII on the leg. The Pope blew a fuse, threw the Cardinal out, and refused to grant Henry his wish—thereby leading to the creation of the Church of England.

I do not expect a church; I just pray that she one day amounts to *something*.

I have read aloud to Willow the story of Bounce, the dog who saved Alexander Pope from a knife-wielding valet, and of Cap, the sheepdog who inspired Florence Nightingale to take up nursing. I have read to her the remarkable tale of Biche, Frederick the Great's beloved

Italian greyhound, who was so valued in battle that, when Biche was captured during the Battle of Soor in 1745, Frederick called it "the kidnapping of a member of the royal family" and arranged a "prisoner exchange" to get the dog back.

I have read to her—sometimes while she sleeps, legs straight up—the story of Peps, who so inspired Wagner when he was at the piano that the great composer once actually claimed that Peps was co-author of *Tannhauser*. (Whether Peps would want such credit is open to speculation.) She has also heard, both while sleeping and awake, the story of Tuck, the Scottish greyhound who stood, and died bravely, fighting with General George Armstrong Custer at the Battle of Little Big Horn.

I have read aloud to her so that she will appreciate the deep connection between great dogs and great men— and if I can still aspire, in my advancing years, to be one of these two, then she should aspire to be the other.

I have told her about the Skye terrier that Alexander Graham Bell taught to say "How are you, Grandmama?" while the little dog growled and Bell manipulated its lips, and I have explained to her how all this led, eventually, to the invention of the machine I sometimes call her on from out of town in the hopes that she will recognize my voice and remember me. I have told her the story of Sigmund Freud and how he would hold birthday parties for his various inspirational dogs, great man and dogs sitting around the table wearing silly paper hats, Freud writing special poems for each dog that he would read aloud with great drama while the dogs checked the meter and rhyme schemes.

We have read together the story of Pat, who some claim was the true prime minister of Canada in the days of William Lyon Mackenzie King. The way things have been going around here lately, I have told Willow, it is not entirely out of the question for her to dream of one day holding higher office.

And, as well, we have read together the stories from Mr. Coren's delightful book on the incredible number of dogs—he estimates 230—who have lived at the White House. She has heard all about Skip, the famous mutt Teddy Roosevelt called "a little dog—by that I mean a little of this, and a little of that." She has listened to the stories of Fala, FDR's little dog who was made a private in the U.S. Army. And, of course, she has heard all about Millie, Barbara Bush's springer spaniel whose major literary effort, *Millie's Book,* actually outsold the president's memoirs.

You would think all this would sink in. But no, I read and she sleeps, and when I stop reading she goes and pokes about under and in the furniture until she finds one of those balls that have been thrown and retrieved so often it looks as though the last time it was thrown was up. She drops it on the open book, sitting back and staring, staring, staring....

# Lost Dog
## at Twenty Below

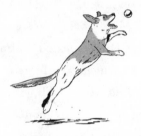

The call came late on the shortest day of the year. It was the youngest, on a cellphone, his voice breathless and thin as if coming from somewhere deep back in the bush—which, in fact, it was.

"Willow's gone!"

He and a pal had taken their dogs—the pal's dog a true border collie, ours a borderline collie with borderline intelligence—off to an area park known on local maps as the Bruce Pit. In local circles, however, it is known as the Dog Convention Centre, a place where mostly purebreds and a few mutts run wild in gangs, a designated sanctuary with not a single sign threatening the dogs with fines if they don't keep their owners on a short leash.

There are, increasingly, such places to be found in Canadian cities. Male dogs arrive convinced that the Supreme Court of Domesticated Animals has declared the entire park a swingers' club; females, as a result, spend much of their time sitting on cold snow and snapping angrily at pestering males; and owners sip coffee—Starbucks snobs in one corner, people with taste in another—and talk about such pressing matters as the best place to find designer pet clothes and debate the benefits of modern crate-training over traditional house-training.

It is hard to believe how the politicians have missed all this. In this country they think there are votes to be had for something as minor as daycare spaces for preschoolers, little realizing that any political party offering to subsidize agility classes for puppies would sweep the country.

The idea in coming to Bruce Pit this bitterly cold day was to "socialize" the dog. She is one year old this month, frighteningly friendly to humans but skittish around other dogs, especially those with loud barks and untoward intentions.

The idea was to let her run with the older, more secure border collie. The two of them could snake about the park in that odd you-can't-see-me slouch of the herding collie, perhaps meet a few regular dogs, and maybe even realize how lucky they are that their owners haven't turned them into fake-fur-and-bootie-wearing Barbie doll dogs.

It worked fine for a while—right up until they happened to run smack into an evolving dog fight over some imagined slight. The little dog bolted immediately. Straight under the dark skirts of the nearest spruce, off back into the deep, deep woods—and gone.

*"Bring warm clothes!"* the youngest shouted into the phone, teeth chattering in the background. *"It's freezing!"*

It was twelve below when we got there. The boy, having headed out in nothing but a fleece, looked like he needed medical attention, not help looking for the lost dog. He put on the ski clothes we had brought along, pulled on thick mittens and a toque, and all of us, some carrying flashlights, headed off deep into the pit.

Darkness fell and the moon, fortunately, rose. It was a bright, clear night, but the advantage given to the eyes came with a disadvantage to the rest of the system: the temperature was now twenty below and heading lower. Up and down the trails we searched, calling her name and, so long as it was still possible to purse lips in such cold, whistling for her. But nothing.

"She won't last more than a couple of hours in this," someone said. No one argued, though no one knew for certain.

The hope that she'd gone elsewhere was really no hope at all. The only exit from the pit parking area was out onto a busy road, the traffic heavy and fast at this time of day, late rush hour, and impossible for a small, frightened dog to get across to where she might find a friendly back door to whine at and scratch on.

After several hours, there was no choice but to give up. No dog and too cold for humans. We arrived home in a stunned, depressed state. A little dog that doesn't have the sense to come in out of the rain was out now in sub-zero temperature, thick bush in one direction, heavy traffic in the other.

Inside the house there was, for once, nothing wiggling and wagging with a shoe in her mouth. There was, however, something. The telephone was flashing red with a message.

A man had been driving home late from work. Traffic on the busy road had come to a halt as a small, skittish dog darted out and then back. He had opened his door, called, and she leapt in—trusting completely in strangers, just as she had been taught.

His wife had tracked us down through Willow's tags. "We have your dog," the message said. She left their number, and then a giggle. "No need to hurry," she added. "She's down in the basement, playing with the children."

But we hurried anyway.

# Merchandising
# Madness

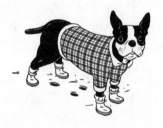

Here, by the front counter, we have a tray of mailman's
fingers—a dollar each. Cheaper, surely, by the gross.
And there, behind the party hats and tutus and faux fur
coats, we find the stack of penises. Bull penises. Bullies.
Pizzle sticks. Whatever you're more comfortable with ...

On the other hand, perhaps it is not so much this
pile of stiff, dried-out bull penises—"an excellent chew
to remove plaque and tarter buildup"—that is causing
the peculiar itching, sweaty feeling that is rippling up
and down your spine as you walk around this high-end

store in the trendiest section of town. Perhaps it is the whole idea.

This store is hardly unique, though it is unusual. It is part of a small chain of dog "boutiques" that go under the Bark & Fitz banner and are amusing stops for the curious as well as treasured stops for the domesticated. There is a bowl of treats at the front entrance and a seemingly endless supply of treats from the small bakery at the back—so long as you come in on all fours with your tail wagging. Dogs, the woman running the shop says, have become "the new children."

Such shifts seem to happen from time to time. Loud men talking on their ear-clip cellphones in busy airports are, most would agree, the new sign of mental illness, as surely as it used to be the goofy guy talking to himself as he walks down the street and makes sure to touch every passing telephone pole.

I was tempted to suggest that dogs have become the new Barbie dolls—something for grownups to dress up and play with using elaborate pretend sets—but then it was pointed out to me that dogs, in fact, now have their own Barbie-like dolls to play with, and so the analogy hardly works. Better just to admit that dogs have become the new children for those who have not yet had their children or, just as often, have had their children and need some replacement to blow their life savings on as they drive themselves increasingly around the bend.

Certainly, the madness applied to the care and raising of dogs has reached heights not even imagined by those who devoted previous years to the care and raising of small humans. The young girl helping out in this shop, for example, is at the computer, trying to register her puppy on some website devoted to purebred Labrador retrievers. She has stalled because she does not have its full identification numbers yet, including the details required for a computer chip that the veterinarian will be embedding between his shoulder blades. This is frustrating to her and, being naturally curious, I ask her how old her puppy is.

"I don't have him yet," she says.

"Oh," I nod, understanding. But, it turns out, not understanding at all.

She continues on: "He won't be born until August—he's not even conceived yet." Planned Parenthood, eat your heart out.

This friendly store is busy and, apparently, prospering. It has a line of fur products—Buddy Wash, Woof, Flip—and even a line of mint pet aromatics devoted to improving the morning breath of your dog: Dewdrop Doggie, Honeysuckle Hound, Bow Wow Bouquet. There are designer clothes, including tuxedos for small dogs. There are dog bath towels with "Stud" stitched on them, little ball caps (with holes for ears) featuring favourite sports teams, party hats, tutus, fake-diamond-encrusted collars, and an entire section dedicated to doggie bling: tiaras, charms to hang from collars, even strings of fake pearls as fat as ping-pong balls.

But this is nothing.

AT THE BIG-BOX BOOKSTORE in the suburbs of this city, there are more publications devoted to pets than to world peace, religion, and philosophy combined. There is a book on petrosexuals, a play on that irritating "metrosexual" word that essentially stands for everything self-centred and, ultimately, meaningless. There is a distinguished-looking "Memory Book" for the assemblage of photographs, anecdotes, tributes, and final collars of the dear departed family pet.

And there are more magazines on dogs than on ... children. *Modern Dog,* for example, has a cover story titled "Britney vs Spot—Trends in Dog Names." It has a feature article on "What to Get the Dog Who Has Everything," another on actress Shannon Elizabeth (one of *Maxim*'s "hottest women in the world"), who says, "My dogs are my kids!", and a third on the art of interviewing potential dog sitters. There are small news items of interest to modern dog owners, including the story—can this possibly be serious?—of a Hindu dog wedding held recently in India for two Labrador retrievers who met through an online doggie dating service. The bride, Diana, is described as looking "ravishing wearing traditional red."

There are ads for $5,000 oil portraits of the family pet, ads for lines of wine—including Pinot Noir and

Chardonnay—that "salute 'man's best friend,'" and page after glossy page of haute couture advertisements for faux fur coats and collars and diamond accessories. High-end hotel chains, including Hilton and Delta, have taken out ads to let potential customers know that their pooches are more than welcome for overnight stays. Whether they get doggie points is not mentioned.

There are also ads for neckties featuring more than seventy-five different breeds. There are pet urns and memorials. There is a special service, Little Lotus Hearts, that provides prayer to ease the mourning of lost pets and even offers to help the distraught sponsor such things as bird and bat houses in the hopes that giving to others might help ease the loss. There are dozens upon dozens of ads for special doggie carrying bags—made famous, presumably, by Paris Hilton and her Chihuahua—including one brand that claims to be "moisture, stain, bacteria and odor resistant."

Most curious of all, however, is a large advertisement for Nintendogs Software, a Nintendo game that lets you research, purchase, and raise a "digital puppy." The game comes in three versions with six available breeds—mutt likely not among them—and is considered the perfect real-puppy replacement therapy for the "high-rise dweller who doesn't relish those regular post-and-plastic bag trips, via the elevator, to the park." And, once your digital puppy is up and running and you're willing to shell out extra for Nintendo's state-of-the-art DS Touch Screen, "you can also pet and rub your puppy's ears."

*New York Dog* seems just a tad brassier, especially when your eye catches the cover stories: "374 Hot Looks," "Desperate House Dogs," and "Is My Dog Bi-Polar?" This magazine is far more into apparel than *Modern Dog,* from leather designer carrying bags to designer paw wear and more bling than Mr. T. would dare wear were he purebred rather than pure ham. "Diamond Dogs," reads one full-page ad from The Gilded Paw, "... when it's more than love."

The most functional-looking collar in the magazine is a specially designed unit to put an end to the lost dog. It has a built-in Global Positioning System so that the owner can track the frisky dog that has caught spring fever and bolted. It has a call-back system for easy use by those who might find the dog, built-in Auto-LED lights for night tracking, and a "Hear Now" two-way radio pet communication with a twelve-mile range for those owners who still feel they can talk some sense into the poor randy beast.

There is also an elaborate glamour photo section showing various celebrities with their dogs: "Carmen Electra and Daisy shopping at Intuition in Hollywood." "Mickey Rourke and Loki on location in London." Hilary Duff, Serena Williams, Sandra Bullock, Uma Thurman, Sharon Osbourne, and Pink are all lovingly photographed with their main pets.

*New York Dog* offers dog horoscopes—Taurus: "The dust settles and you have survived a domestic storm. You can come out from hiding"—as well as a pet psychologist's advice column called "On the Couch," which in older days was the last place in the world the dog was allowed. And where the psychologist comes up short, the "Psychic Companion" columnist steps in. Shown nothing but photographs of, for example, a hugely missed dead dog, the psychic is able to offer remarkable comfort: "I picked up that he was deeply connected to your spirit, and has been so for centuries."

When it comes to advertisements, *New York Dog* is in a class by itself: edible gingerbread homes for dogs, temporary tattoos for dogs—"Dogs Rule! Cats Suck!"— and even pet jewellery for the owners, including a $1,200 14k gold bracelet with five charms specific to your pet.

There are fashion pages featuring fully dressed animals wearing the same insouciant, world-weary look that supermodels affect. There are more shots of the famous with their dogs—Princess Grace, Barbara Bush, Nancy Reagan, Martha Stewart—and there is, most unexpected of all, page after page, complete with colour photographs, of obituaries sent in by bereaved families, the pet every bit as lovingly remembered as—perhaps more so than—grandma herself.

Ol' Yeller, one suspects, would pull the trigger himself if he were still around.

# Dogs as Fashion Accessories

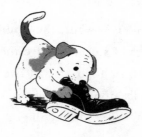

It was not, I can assure you, an acid flashback. There it was, on channel seven, a dog that had not been seen since shortly after Jim Morrison took up permanent residence in Paris, since Pierre and Margaret were together and having Christmas babies, since it seemed the entire world, not just this particular dog breed, had long and silky hair.

An Afghan.

It was riding in the back seat of something called an Optra, a new Chevrolet that is being flogged as "sleek and stylish," and the dog, presumably, had been placed in the commercial to demonstrate just that—as well as to make a corny joke about sunroofs and the tangled, windblown hair that some of us, long, long ago, once enjoyed.

I sat there wondering where they found the dog. I have not seen an Afghan since, oh, around 1975, when the street we lived on in Toronto had five and they seemed as momentarily fashionable as leisure suits and quadraphonic sound. Where did they all go?

Dogs were fashion accessories long before Paris Hilton went in search of a Chihuahua small enough to fit in her makeup kit. Afghans somewhat superseded the Irish setter, and soon enough both breeds—perhaps given up on by owners tired of spending all their free time cutting out burrs—gave way to a fad that wasn't even a breed at all but rather the strange art of "puppy repackaging."

There was a time when, if someone had a poodle that went into heat and took off on the lam with the neighbourhood spaniel, the owner of the female would simply deal with the consequences of that lapse of judgment—or, more accurately, lapse of backyard fence. Weeks would pass, perhaps a couple of months, and the owner now of several dogs would pay whatever it cost to put a small ad in the local paper saying "Puppies: poodle and spaniel mix, free to good home."

But no longer.

What the pet stores started to do—no one knows exactly where this devious practice began—was take that poodle running off with that spaniel and turn their natural byproduct into brand-new faux "breed," which they then flog for the price of a used car. Once pet stores discovered that whatever came of that poodle and spaniel dalliance could be marketed as "spoodles," the entire dog world underwent a paradigm shift in common sense. Soon there were cockapoos and terripoos—and, for all we know, Great Poos—until today there are nearly two dozen "poo" mixes available. Which only goes to prove that a poodle running loose is even looser than anyone ever imagined.

The falling in and out of dog fashion was all brought home when a recent issue of *Country Life*, the rather snooty British leisure magazine, ripped into readers for choosing certain colonial dog breeds—the Nova Scotia duck tolling retriever and the Labrador retriever—over homegrown breeds. Canadian dogs, it seems, are suddenly hot. We have only four "recognized" breeds, and here were two of them on the list of most popular dogs in Great Britain, which everyone knows is the pet-loving centre of the universe.

The tolling retriever I am not familiar with—they apparently have the ability to attract ducks and, oddly, Scandinavia has more of these dogs than North America does—but the Labrador retriever is, of course, familiar to all. Labs are, in fact, the most popular registered dog in the world, according to most lists released by the various kennel clubs.

The German shepherd usually runs second or third in such lists, but the British are apparently in a dither over the fading popularity of such standard fare as the cocker spaniel and the bull terrier. The bull terrier has had its reputation somewhat shaken, however, by Princess Anne's two bull terriers, Dotty and Flo, and their predilection for attacking small children, corgis, and maids' knees.

No one fully understands what makes a breed popular one decade while it vanishes the next. Labs are easygoing and great with children, which explains their continuing popularity, but the Chihuahua seems to have popped up on the lists in response to Paris Hilton and Taco Bell ads. And not that long ago, the Jack Russell terrier was enjoying a popularity that could be directly attributed to the *Frasier* television show and its endless reruns.

I asked a friend who is a vet where the Afghan went, and he wasted few words in explaining its quick demise: not particularly smart, not particularly good with children, and too time-consuming to groom. "What I'd really like to know," he said after summarily dismissing the poor Afghan, "is where did the standard collie go? You know, the Lassie dog—I hardly ever see one any more."

Nor have I, come to think of it. And yet there was a time when Lassie was Hollywood's greatest star, appearing in movies with everyone from Elizabeth Taylor to Jimmy Stewart. The dogs were everywhere, big and friendly and as much a symbol of the happy suburban family as the Lab is today. "Great dogs," said the vet. "Great, great dogs."

But the best dog, for his money, might be the one dog that has the least to do with money: the mutt.

The mutt was once the only fashion—roughly separated into one group for work, one for hunting, one for hanging around—and it was only when the middle class began springing up and looking for anything that might translate into a little more social status that the poor mutt began having trouble finding its place. Having the "right" dog was just one more trapping.

And if you think it's tough being a mutt in today's world, just think about what it was like back in Britain when the push for proper "breeds" began. There was even, at one point, an anti-mutt movement during the late Victorian era of the 1890s, with one famous commentator on animal care telling Brits, "No one would plant weeds in a flower garden, so why have mongrels as pets?"

Well, I must confess here to having had an incredible string of them. And proud of it. The current one, Bandit, is going on fourteen, is stiff and deaf, but has never suffered from hip dysplasia and other assorted genetic conditions that seem to afflict so many expensive breeds. She is also excellent with children and alarming to burglars. Same for the previous mutt, who cost nothing and lived sixteen years. And the one before that, who also happily lived to a ripe old age. "Your next dog," says one daughter, speaking like a car salesman trying to fit us into a minivan, "has to be a Portuguese water dog."

No thanks. I not only have no idea what they are, I don't care. Besides, what would happen if they suddenly go out of fashion like the poor Afghan? It's mutts for me, as it should be for all people—who are, if you think about it, themselves mutts of a fashion.

# Squirrels
# and Sisyphus

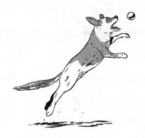

Bark!

(*Bark!*)

Bark! Bark!

(*Bark! Bark!*)

Bark! Bark! Bark!

(*Bark! Bark! Bark!*)

"It's your echo, idiot!"

She pays no heed. Bark! Bark! (*Bark! Bark!*)

It happens several times a day. This time it was a woodpecker that set her off. A while back, a squirrel.

Last night, a barred owl. She barks, another dog instantly answers. It does not seem to occur to her that each bark is identical to the other, that they are bouncing back from across the bay. Even if I shout—"Shut up!" (*"Shut up!"*)—it doesn't seem to register with her that there is absolutely nothing across the water, just a high hill and an echo.

Willow and I have come here to this isolated northern lake to try to undo all that has taken place over the past few months as this poor mutt suffers through the petification of North American society.

Having taken total control of their children's lives, having sucked childhood dry of happenstance and idle time, those whose children have moved on and those whose children have yet to come have turned their astounding micromanaging skills on their dogs. When the pet stores are larger than Wal-Mart, you have a problem. When they serve the puppy first at the Tim Hortons window, you have a problem.

This dog has more toys than any of the four children who previously passed through these doors. She has one diploma and is currently working on a second, which at the current rate will shortly give her more formal education than her master. *Master*—now there's a word that has lost all meaning....

No matter, with dog classes done for the week and no appearance of homework—I mean, how many times can you be told to sit and wait for a green street light you never noticed in the first place?—I decided to take the mutt and head up to the lake and let her learn for herself some of life's great lessons. Like, no matter how quick you are, no matter how high you lunge, you will never, ever, catch a squirrel. And don't poke that wet nose too close to the fireplace.

The learning curve here at the lake is so different, in fact, from the world she lives in the rest of the time that I have taken the liberty of assigning a few marks and comments:

### BUGS: D−

It is not possible, no matter how many diplomas or degrees this dog ultimately ends up with, to leap into the air and snap every single mosquito and blackfly and deer fly to death. On the other hand, this may be the first time in history that a dog has been exercised daily by a swarm of insects. It can't be long before the pet super-store starts selling portable "bug rooms" to keep city dogs as sharp and active as dogs at the lake.

### RESPECT FOR THE DEAD: F

In the city, this mostly white-furred creature loves nothing better than to roll about in clean snow or a freshly cut lawn. Here, she has so far rolled on a dead squirrel, a crushed shrew, and some fish guts illegally and ignorantly left near the government landing by some intruder. An F also goes to the human who forgot to bring the ridiculous crate she sleeps in at home, which means that her now-rancid coat has left its delightful scent all over the bed.

### NATURE STUDIES: D+

The dogwood is in full bloom and glorious. She has not even noticed. She has discovered, on the other hand, that rotten wood chews more easily than green hard-wood and that there is nothing quite so cool, after some hot running, as lying down in the mud by the little creek.

### FAUNA RECOGNITION: F−

On the drive in, we passed two small moose standing by the side of the road and one otter that ran across directly in front of the vehicle. She noticed nothing. Let a squirrel even tick a tiny paw nail while creeping about the property, however, and she is off like a heat-seeking missile. She has no sense, obviously, that they are the ones in charge of this endless game.

### FETCHING: A+

We spent much of Saturday down by the landing, me tossing sticks in and imploring her to act like a proper dog. She watched several fly out and splash, and then she went off in search of more fish guts to roll in. Finally, she returned, calmly swam out to where one stick was still floating, brought it in, and dropped it by my feet.

I, of course, threw it again. She, sensibly, shook off the ice-cold water—once is enough!—and darted off in search of something less predictable than a human.

BARK! BARK!

*(Bark! Bark!)*

"Come back here!"

*("Come back here!")*

It occurs to me, in moments like this, that there may be more difference between the city dog and the country dog than we realize. Especially when we are speaking of what we take to be the same dog, merely in different locales. I used to think the lake was a place where we went to escape the real world. But now I realize that it might well be another world. Or more accurately, a parallel universe, a never-discovered dimension, an alternative reality where nothing is as it was in the world just fled.

The dog at home is pure routine: she sleeps in a crate and is wagging her tail before seven, when the first one up comes downstairs. She scoops up a dirty sock or old sneaker, wiggles wildly, races up the stairs, and jumps, paws first, onto the head of the one still sleeping. She then goes outside, briefly, always tied to a line, and returns instantly upon completion of the tasks at paw. She curls up on a mat and sleeps most of the morning, moving only to bark at the mail dropping into the outside box. At noon she places a heavy head on my knee and stares. It is time for the walk. The long walk completed, she goes back to sleep, usually upside down with all four paws in the air. At 3:45 sharp, she comes back into the office with a lacrosse ball in mouth and makes enough of a nuisance repeatedly dropping it on the hardwood floor that I get up and take her to the field for a half hour of fetch. She goes back to bed. She gets out again late and then goes, usually on her own, off to her crate for the night. (We live in Ottawa. So you're welcome to think of this little dog, Willow, as the animal version of a civil servant.)

For a long time I believed it was this dog we were taking to the lake. Same colour, same size, answers—sometimes—to the same name. But I now see that it is another dog entirely.

The dog that is at the lake has no routine. She begins to dance the moment the packing begins. The instant the vehicle turns onto the first back road, she transforms into a furry creature that makes the Energizer bunny seem like a stuffed animal. By the time the tires hit gravel, she is virtually steering.

The dog that sleeps all day at home hardly sleeps at all at the lake. From dawn to midnight, she chases squirrels, sniffs through the woods, and pounds the outside of the screen door with sticks, dropping them only if someone is foolish enough to answer. She then backs off, crouching low in the hopes that the person will take pity on her and try—I dare you!—to throw the stick of the moment where it cannot be retrieved.

At home she is so clean the kids will often bury their faces in her fur; at the cottage that fur often needs burying itself. At home, she sleeps in her crate; at the cottage she lies where she wishes. At home, she takes a back seat; at the cottage, she moves instantly to the front of the boat, hanging off the bow like Kate Winslet in *Titanic*.

I suppose, however, that this parallel universe for pets really should come as no great surprise. After all, when you think about it, it applies to us as well. The difference is, when I sleep through the winter, I don't dream of chasing squirrels at the lake. And I don't stick my legs straight up in the air, churning madly. At least no one has ever mentioned it.

# In the Now
# of Mid-life

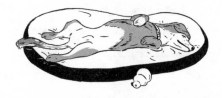

"What," the question goes, "does a man do standing up that a woman does sitting down that a dog does on three legs?"

"Shake hands."

That was my first off-colour joke, told to me at age six or seven. Since those long-ago days I have grown up—if only somewhat—but I still puzzle over the many differences and similarities between humans and their pets. In some ways it all depends on perspective: as the old saying goes, they drink out of our toilet, we pee in their water bowl. But still, there is one pressing matter that has one telling answer.

Question: "What do most men go through that no dog ever does?"

Answer: "A mid-life crisis."

Man in mid-life—or so I hear—is often at his worst: insecure, unhappy, confused, uncertain, desperate to be anything but what he is at this precise moment. A dog in mid-life, on the other hand, lives in the moment— and could not possibly be happier.

The dog does not pine for those days when it got in trouble for piddling on the floor, or for that day when it went off in the car to that awful place with the cold steel tabletops and came out a couple of days later without its reproductive organs. Nor is the dog filled with regret for paths not taken—largely because it took them all. It does not lament dead gophers not rolled in or bums not sniffed. It does not mourn for those missed golden opportunities when the collar suddenly snapped off and, for a moment, the entire world was calling out to have its territory marked off.

At night, dogs don't stare at their reflections in the sliding doors and wonder if their fur is thinning. They don't nervously pop little breath mints—though it *would* be nice. Most of them—especially yellow Labs—seem to take enormous pride in their love handles. And the very notion of their ever needing a special pill to hop the leg of the first stranger coming in through the front door is simply preposterous.

Dogs in mid-life are in their prime. They are healthy, wise, content, and the greatest companion possible. They are, simply, what we see when we think of dogs. Puppies can capture your heart; old dogs will break your heart; but it is the mid-life dog that owns your heart.

It's something about dependability, I guess. The best dog name I ever came across is in Wayland Drew's poetic *Halfway Man,* a novel about Native and white values colliding north of Lake Superior. Travis Niskigwun has the greatest dog imaginable: a big middle-aged mutt who is always by his side, always ready to do his slightest bidding.

The dog's name? "Guaranteed."

Not all of my dogs reached middle age. The first, as I have mentioned before, was only a puppy when hit by a garbage truck; the most recent is still a young adult. But Cindy, Bumps, and Bandit all had glorious and healthy years when they were simply "the dog," by far the most dependable, and likely the most universally beloved, member of the entire family.

Guaranteed.

Something eventually happens to a dog as he or she grows into middle age. One day the leash, which you had previously needed to hang on to as you would a rope tow at a ski hill, suddenly goes slack, a welcome and telling bow between the human hand that holds it and the collar where it is attached. In some cases the leash is no longer even necessary, but is needed, curiously, by dog as much as by owner—almost as if it is walking you, not the other way around.

Bandit, curiously, was comfortable during walks only if she held a part of the leash in her mouth, just to be sure the human was coming along at Bandit's chosen pace. After I put the leash on I had to fold it back and allow her to chomp down on the hand loop, and then off we'd go, the walker hopping along beside her on a very short leash indeed.

One day, somewhat beyond the second year, it becomes possible to let the dog out the back door and it does not run away but sits, patiently, waiting for you to put on your boots and perhaps even your jacket, hat, and gloves and come and enjoy the fresh air. One day, for no apparent reason, the grown dog can take or leave a thrown ball. One day, for no reason at all, it stops racing along the paths with a massive stick in the mouth, clipping the shins and calves of every human foolish enough to think the traffic will show courtesy. One day there is no longer a dirty sock or an old shoe in the mouth.

And so begins the very best time of your relationship, that long stretch when, if I may be permitted a little human vanity here, owner and pet are equals, the relationship symbiotic—they need us to feed them; we need them to greet us—and as comfortable and, truly, as rich as or richer than any other friendship you will ever make.

I may not know art, but I know what I like—and I love what the eccentric Vincent Van Gogh once had to say about the art of owning a canine pet: "If you don't have a dog—at least one—there is not necessarily anything wrong with you, but there may be something wrong with your life." Again, guaranteed.

Each mature dog is, of course, different. When Cindy was middle-aged and I was a teenager we lived in a small town in Central Ontario, and the best parts were the long hikes up through the woods behind Reservoir Hill and chasing sticks out well past the big floating dock at my grandparents' log home in Algonquin Park. When Bumps was middle-aged and I was in my twenties and thirties, there were still small children for her to spend hours rounding up and making sure they didn't wander off. She was child, sibling, and even parent to all six of us humans in the various houses in which we lived as we moved about the province. When Bandit was middle-aged and I was well into my forties and early fifties, the kids began moving out to go away to school and she was the constant comfort that made their leaving somewhat acceptable and, more importantly, made their returns home moments of great barking and wiggling joy.

Willow is the first dog I have beaten to middle age. It is both an amusing and an alarming thought. I never expected to grow up so quickly. Yet now I am wanting Willow to grow up too quickly, it seems, just so that she can become that remarkable, constant sidekick that a middle-aged dog becomes, a presence so natural and easy that it is remarked upon only when it is gone.

Journalists don't have mid-life crises. We have mid-year, mid-month, mid-week, and even mid-day crises. (There, I just had one mid-sentence!) I am not as comfortable in my own skin as any dog I have had is, but I expect that is merely a human condition. Dogs know exactly who they are and haven't the slightest interest in the question; humans waste a good portion of their lives on questions that have no answers.

What dogs do—particularly a middle-aged, confident, contented dog—is offer perspective. They can cause you to look at something from another angle, to realize, in an instant, how lucky you are and how foolish you've been. Kids do much the same, especially when they are very young and don't know what it is you do for a living, let alone care about your work and the enormous weight you allow it to place on your shoulders. Travel gives a different and equally welcome perspective, distance and time away making those things you take for granted— from your own backyard to your own country—suddenly seem special, as if you'd somehow failed to take proper notice and appreciate.

Travel, however, far too quickly recedes. Kids change, as they should, from treating you as the centre of their lives to wanting you at the furthest fringes of their lives to, eventually, accepting and even embracing you as a significant part of their lives. The dog, on the other hand, never seems to change, not even when the end is near. Your coming through that front door remains, right to final tail wag, the single most significant event in the history of that moment—for the moment is all that they live for. And living for the moment is the secret that they give to us.

Today we went walking, as usual, down by the creek. It was snowing lightly, winter clearly getting its directions

confused, but the spring melt from the previous day
had the creek brown and swollen and as inviting to the
one-year-old dog as a warm bath might be to an eighty-
year-old human.

My mood fit the mood of the day, overcast and
downcast. Word the previous night at hockey had been
that one of the longtime players is battling cancer. A
man only into his forties, a gifted athlete with a young
family, hit hard by that one attacker so difficult to turn
back. Word had also come that an old neighbour had
passed on, a funny Scot who owned a Scottie and who
had no children of his own, but, with his wonderful
wife, took on the children from all sides of the street to
the point where the children thought of them as "spare"
grandparents.

One can only slip down so deep in one's thoughts
when a dog is around. She raced about, trying to break
branches off from trees, until I pulled my sorry hands
out of my pockets and broke one off for her and threw
it. And threw it again. And threw it again. And again
and again and again.

We walked for more than an hour. She scared herself half to death by bolting over a bank and practically landing on a couple of mallards that exploded from the water. She almost got stuck in a gopher hole. She ran and ran and ran, and then ran some more, her fur soaked through with creek water, streaked with mud, never happier because, to her, there is no never. Only now.

I talk a lot to her, just as I have to all the other dogs. It's a strange, one-way conversation, quite different from any you might have with, say, a baby or a toddler who also does not understand whatever language you are using. I talk to the dog about what we're doing, what we're seeing, sometimes even what we're thinking. Or at least what one of us is thinking. She couldn't care less.

She cares only about the walk, the water, the sticks, the throwing, the smells, the sounds. She has been this way since she was a puppy and she will be this way right to her final walk down along this creek, a walk in which only one of us will return with a heavy heart. But that is a long, long, long way off. Perhaps by then we will both be in old age.

Right now she clears away the internal clouds with her running and her jumping and her foolishness—"Get your head out of that hole!"—and in her sheer, open delight at doing nothing but hanging out with you in a place both of you love. That is the essence of the middle-aged dog she will eventually become: a welcome companion, no matter what you might be doing or what might be on your mind. Perspective, delivered daily.

I would never suggest that dogs offer a superior perspective on life than children do, just a slightly different one. Both tell you that there are far more important things in life than what you might have on your mind. But there are differences. If you show up at your front door having been fired over lunch by the boss, the children will want to know how it affects them; the dog will want to know when you are going for the walk together.

Those walks—down by the creek one day, through the woods the next, around the block if it's raining hard— are, for many of us, a critical salvation in life. The dog is interested only in getting going. He or she lives absolutely in the moment—the most important thing in the world being the sound of the leash coming down, then the most important thing in the world the door, then the most important thing in the world trying to figure out what other dog came and peed on this tire or that snowbank. Simple, yes, but an astounding and absolutely welcome simplicity after a tough day as a human.

There is simply no *down* to dog. She has just come to me with a new stick and, when I try to take it from her, she hangs on so tightly that I am able to lift her entirely off the ground, swinging her around and around and around until stick snaps and dog goes flying, bouncing straight back for more of the same. I'm sure dog disciplinarians would frown on such activity, but this, surely, is more a case of the dog dealing with the human than the human with the dog. If I felt down moments earlier, now I am roaring with laughter, near tears at the absurdity of this new game she has invented on the spot.

I cannot say it as accurately or as well as James Thurber—"Dogs are *obsessed* with being happy"—so I won't even bother trying. I'll just enjoy. And be thankful for all those years of being welcomed at the front door by someone who knows what really and truly matters in life.

Tummy scratches.

What a dog does on its back and a man does leaning down.

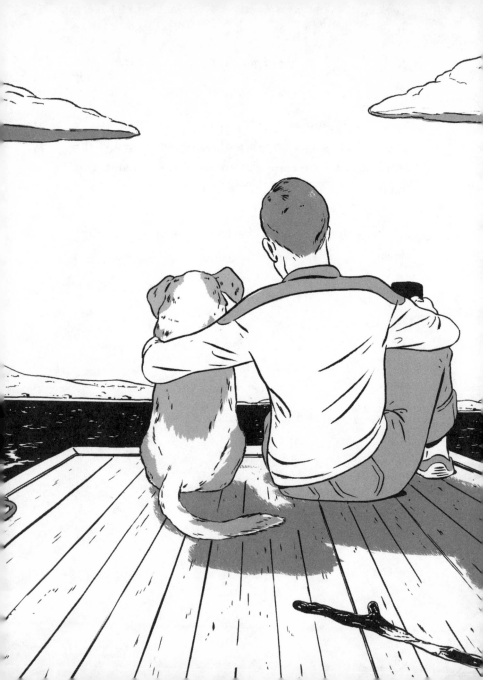

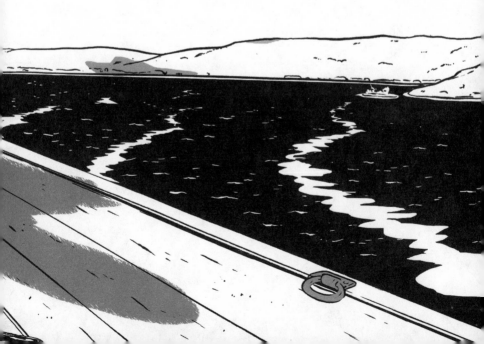
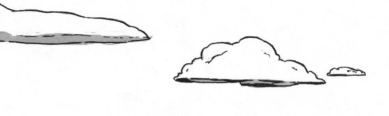

So Very Old

# Dog in Winter

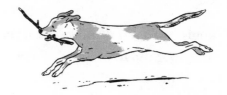

It snowed during the night, huge flakes that fell so slowly it seemed they were drifting through water. By morning it was clear that—in this particular part of this vast country, anyway—we shall have that white, politically correct holiday time of year everyone craves.

The old dog, Bandit, noticed the second she was let out for the morning. Instead of heading to the end of her chain to do her usual duty, she stepped out into the deep fluff, suddenly reared back on her back legs like Silver at the end of a *Lone Ranger* episode, and lunged, literally lunged off the back deck as if she were diving into warm summer water rather than the form water takes in winter in these parts.

It is December and it is white. The world is as it should be. November, the one month most Canadians would vote off the calendar, is gone with its blowing leaves, wet winds, and early evenings so dark not even a flashlight cares to go out in them. Soon it will be January, the month that seems to take up too much of the Canadian calendar, but for now there is fresh snow on the ground, and everyone, even this old dog romping in the backyard, feels a bit like the children let out for recess in the nearby schoolyard, running and leaping and laughing as if the snow were something to swim in and eat at the same time, a great unexpected surprise that somehow fell out of the sky in the night.

The snow is above the ankle but below the knee, a far cry from the four storeys of snow that have already been dumped on the Maritimes, and it is, for the moment, still a joy to shovel. I head out with Bandit, she plowing her nose through the fallen cover as if, somehow, it helps. It doesn't, of course, but it still looks as if we are working together.

A neighbour down the street has a snow blower. In December I stand on the drive, scraper in hand, praying he will not offer to help out; by February I will stand by the window, coffee in hand, praying he will beat me to it and do the obvious neighbourly thing.

I number among the millions for whom the snow shovel is the only household tool we have ever mastered. That clean walk, that squared-off drive is the only time in our pathetic lives when we can point to anything we have completed without hitting our thumbs, stripping a screw, or bumping our heads. It is also—though it hardly equals a new cedar deck or a refinished basement—the only visible, albeit temporary, evidence of accomplishment we are ever able to present to the rest of the world.

There was once a time when Canadians were hypersensitive about their dominant season. In the late nineteenth century, British prime minister William Gladstone dismissed us as the land of "perpetual ice and snow," and the Irish newspaper, *The Nation,* ridiculed the place so many Irish were headed for as nothing less than "a kind of Siberia."

At one point, long before political correctness worried about the inadvertent mention of "Christmas," the Canadian government, in its infinite wisdom, ordered that the word "cold" be avoided in all government brochures and publications and be replaced with the far more acceptable word "buoyant." If I were to say to the neighbour, "Buoyant out today, eh?" I would get a look like the dog gives me when I tell her it's time to head back inside.

There was another point when Canadians actually tried to pretend we had no white stuff to speak of here during the "winter" months. When railway magnate William Van Horne used to head off to Europe in search of new investors for his railways and new immigrants to ride them west, he would fake a chill no matter what city he might be in, moaning for all to hear, "How I pine for Winnipeg to thaw me!" I understand he was in Florence the day he said this.

Mercifully, Canadians eventually came to celebrate winter, even trying to sell it to the rest of the world as something that was, indeed, buoyant to the spirit.

Few of us care for so much of it, and almost all of us will be begging, come late February, for it to finally stop snowing, but at the moment it is most welcome. For reasons that no one can understand—any more than we can figure out why the snow the plow deposits at the end of the drive is 2,426 times as dense as the fluff the dog and I are supposed to be shovelling—that first snowfall seems to warm us up as much as it, most assuredly, brightens the evening enough that a flashlight isn't necessary.

Bandit understands this best. The snow seems to have taken a half-century of dog years off her, and she runs as if she would love to be, if it were only possible, both under the snow and on top of it at the same time. What she smells in that fresh snow is unknown; it is, however, delightful to see that nose poking, for once, in a place where I would happily poke my own.

The driveway done, the old dog and I head out for a walk down past the houses and under a roadway to a park where an open creek still churns and defies icing solid, at least for a few more weeks. The scene is sweeter than any of the politically correct holiday-time-of-year cards that have been filling up the mailbox each morning. Deep snow covers the deer trails, falls off into the creek, and flows like slush floes down past the beaver chews and, eventually, into the Ottawa River.

Around one turn the dog suddenly starts, frightened by five mallards that burst from the creek and, in a fury of duck talk and slapping wings, head out over the cornfields on a bearing that will take them south. Perhaps they stayed around just long enough to see winter's exquisite arrival. Perhaps they have already seen enough.

# Grizzled and on the Lam

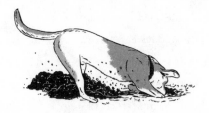

It is always disconcerting to discover that the voice at the other end of the telephone line belongs to the police. And all the more so to learn that they are calling about one of yours.

"We have your dog here at the station."

For a long moment I am speechless, and the Ontario Provincial Police constable mistakes the silence for denial. He recites the numbers of a licence, but they mean nothing. I have never heard those numbers before. Nor, of course, have I ever looked at them.

"It's registered in your name, sir."

I'm sure it is—but still I am speechless.

"Female. Black and brown with a little white, fairly small—is that yours, sir?"

It certainly sounds like her, but how? Bumps is nearly fourteen years old and has not only never before crossed the law, but these days can barely cross the lawn. It would seem more reasonable if the police were calling about one of the kids being caught in a bank holdup, or if our aging Ford Pinto station wagon had turned itself in as a menace to public safety. But we are speaking here of the totally harmless, a mongrel that came from up a street we lived on in Toronto it seems now so very, very long ago.

She was a puppy back then and came to the door in a wagon pulled by neighbourhood kids trying to unload an unwanted litter, and we took one in one of those weak moments that seem to follow puppies around like paper towels. The vet was diplomatic. "I wouldn't expect much if I were you." We did not and were pleasantly surprised. If anything the dog was too dependable.

All dogs are special, but there is something very special about the dog that grows most with your children. It is not about type, but about time—and Bumps's time happily coincided with the time of our own litter: four children, three girls and a boy, spaced out over a mere six years. The first arrived when Bumps was three, and the dog handled the newborn coming home from the hospital far better than any of the children who followed did of the children who followed them. A dog of endless patience—with the peculiar exception of preferring that a child not grab her luxuriant tail—and a dog committed, almost obsessively, to ensuring that none of them, like wayward lambs, ever strayed very far, whether from the backyard or from the shallow end of the dock.

Like everyone's dog, this one had certain special traits—including a strange ability to remove peanuts from the shell and a penchant for ripe raspberries plucked fresh from the bush—but still, just a dog.

After fourteen years, you take them for granted. No one ever notices that the puppy who was once gagging on the end of a leash has not broken away on her own for more than a decade. Everyone else seems to grow after a while, but not the dog. The dog never changes. Or at least you hope. Others, over time, start to see things a bit differently. The vet looks at the old dog and mentions a grizzled mouth or cloudy eyes, but you see only the pup who first came knocking at the door. But then, one day, you are forced to acknowledge what time, curse its hide, has done to your pup.

For this particular dog, it happened recently on a long walk through the woods to an abandoned farm the kids are convinced they can buy and fix up for less than forty cents. Halfway in, the dog lay down panting and simply refused to move. The only way to get her across the mile or so still to cover was to carry her like a baby, which of course I did.

When we reached the farmhouse I carried her inside in search of shade, unfortunately walking straight into a large porcupine coming down the gutted stairwell. Porcupine and person both panicked, but all the dog did was turn slightly in my arms, bark twice, and growl, baring teeth the vet says are desperately in need of scaling. The porcupine also ran for the door but the person, fortunately, won, still carrying the dog like a baby. As I bolted over the broken doors, she tucked her head under my arm and snarled back as if she, somehow, was the one with the porcupine on the run. Perhaps from her perspective it seemed that way. After all, her legs never moved and the porcupine did indeed fade quickly into the distance. The dog had obviously won the day.

Against the porcupine, but not against time. Not against the one enemy that won't be halted by a nasty snarl and the baring of old teeth.

Following that collapse in the woods, it was clear that no one expected much any more. Everyone agreed that fourteen years was a long time—ninety-eight, the more mathematical kids said, in dog years—and from that moment on she was treated as if her glory days were forever gone. After that sad day in the woods, no one even suggested another walk.

"Sir?" It was the voice on the telephone again. The OPP officer. The police calling about the dog.

"Yes—yes, the dog's mine, all right. I'll be right down."

I drove down and parked behind the station. She was sitting at the back near the garage doors, two young officers sitting with her, both with a hand ruffling up and down her back.

"She's never run away before?" the younger officer asked.

"Never."

"Well, we found her running along the road up there. Shaking like a leaf."

"Never seen a dog so nervous," the other officer said. "I wonder what got into her?"

"I don't know," I said.

But later, watching her dance in the seat on the way home, I did know. It wasn't nervousness, but excitement. And what got into her was what should get into us all when they write us off before our time.

# You Will Know
# When It's Time

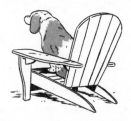

"You will know when it's time."

Fine, but how? There is no expiry date on her that I can find, nothing at all to indicate shelf life apart from the obvious fact that she was clearly "best before" any of this current state of affairs came along. There is no timely reminder in the mail, no message on the answering machine, no waiter discreetly laying her plastic credit card on the table and whispering that it is no longer considered "active." She would take offence to that. She thinks herself very active indeed.

Mercifully, she does not see herself as we have lately seen her.

It is fall now, and this is approximately the sixth time since May that we have come here to the lake together so that Bandit can spend her final days where she has always been happiest. Over those few months, the changes have been dramatic.

I now carry Bandit to the car, place her in a back seat specifically set up so she cannot fall off and get stuck anywhere—and yet several times each drive I will have to stop and adjust her. One time it will be her back legs stuck between seat and door; another time she will be wedged head first between back seat and front seat.

It is foolish for me to be embarrassed for her. She never says a thing about any of this. Of course, it has been a year now since she last barked. Hard to believe, that, since it was always her wild, excited barking that announced we were here, the way others on the lake might hoist a flag.

What is totally mysterious is how this old dog, who cannot see, who cannot hear, still manages to wobble to her four feet when the car turns onto the long country road that leads in here, and how the panting that would have been described as "laboured" only hours earlier is now almost puppylike.

"You will know when it's time." They all say that. And surely, I thought when we headed out, this will be it. There is a shovel leaning against the cabin. There is a special place chosen, back up in the bush by a huge rock that this mutt could once bound onto in a single leap. Now, however, she needs to be carried from the cabin down the three small steps to a flat bit of ground where she awkwardly does the required business and then needs carrying back up again. I do this happily.

I used to be baffled by stories such as the one about legendary hockey coach Roger Neilson pushing his old mutt around in a shopping cart because the dog could no longer walk and Roger simply could not do what needed to be done. But now I understand.

Fifteen years ago, when this mutt was a puppy, we bought a cage that resembled a shopping cart without wheels. The idea was to place the dog in it when we went out. The first time we did go out after the arrival of this old dog as a puppy, we came home and found all four kids inside the cage with the puppy happily bouncing off it as she tried to get at them. They just didn't want to deal with her frenetic energy. Now they have to deal with her lack of energy and are also happy to carry her up and down the steps, more than willing to pick her up when she falls. It's nothing, absolutely nothing, compared with what we all owe her.

The end of a pet is one of the great curiosities of society. Within the family walls, it is devastating. One step beyond those walls it means little. Two steps beyond those walls, it means nothing.

I never expected her to last this long. She wouldn't make the May 24th weekend ... she wouldn't make Canada Day ... she wouldn't make Labour Day ... and now we say she won't make Thanksgiving. But summer did not come to this part of the country until early fall—just as the sixties didn't reach Canada until some time in the early seventies—and so here she still is, still sniffing around the pine needles, still heading instinctively down toward the water. Only with such a difference. Whereas once it was full bore down the hill and off the end of the dock, now it might be slipping and rolling down the hill and falling in.

It helps to remember that this old dog called Bandit— now so skinny, now so helpless—was once the talk of the lake as she was known to swim entirely across it if she heard children swimming, the only sight her barking black and white head and the wake from the powerful strokes that were taking her to the far shore to round up kids.

"You will know when it's time."

I suppose this is true enough. We knew when it was time the last time this situation had to be faced. And the time before that. It's never nice, but one day it simply becomes time.

The lake is remarkably calm, unlike the man standing at the end of the dock wondering what to do, and when to do it. The old dog is at the steps, determined. She locks the back legs that no longer seem to work and hops once, slipping but holding, hops again and is down on her own, blindly heading into a world of a thousand nasal delights. There is, perhaps unintentionally, also a slight bounce to her step. And perhaps the man at the end of the dock misreads it. But so what?

It is not time yet. Not yet.

# Walking Alone

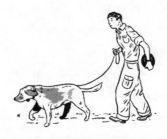

I am having to learn to walk all over again.

Don't misunderstand. I did not break a leg. There is no apparent brain malfunction, despite all those years of covering hockey. I am learning to walk alone, and it is not an easy thing to do. There is no longer a dog around here to walk me (yes, it was finally "time"; enough said, please), and yet I remain one of those people who must, absolutely must, get out each day and work off excess energy.

Writing is a most unusual lifestyle in that you tend to run a marathon each day from the bellybutton up, but do next to nothing from the butt down. For balance—we're talking health here, not journalism—you need to get out and get mobile, whether on a bike or on your own two feet, in whatever fashion they prefer to move. And the beauty of having a dog, even a very old dog, is that the dog gets you out no matter what the weather, no matter what the mood.

For nearly sixteen years Bandit walked me. And for sixteen years before Bandit came along, Bumps walked me. Dogs, in fact, have been walking me since I was eleven years old and a family down by the river was handing out mutts that were still hanging off their one mother but looked as though they had several dozen fathers. So it has been only in these past few weeks that I have realized I cannot walk alone.

When I head down the street and over the crosswalk toward the park we always walked in, I now think every driver passing by figures I have a heart condition. I am out here, walking, under doctor's orders. Or perhaps I am something never before seen in this suburban neighbourhood—a middle-aged man without a car—and am therefore immediately under suspicion.

It has all brought home the fact that we are defined by the company we keep. There is not a man alive who has ever pushed a stroller and not noted how, miraculously, women coming in the other direction no longer avoid eye contact but smile widely at you. And there is not a dog walker born who has not benefited from the doubt that is erased in the minds of all he passes. If the dog is friendly— and all of ours have been tail-wagging, crotch-nuzzling, face-licking basket cases—then the owner is automatically presumed friendly as well, and the strangers will nod and say hello and often even stop to pat a head until they are so soaked in saliva they must head off in search of towels.

I would always end this old dog's walk with a shortcut that brought us back alongside a schoolyard. If we came at noon or recess, we would be instantly surrounded.

"Can I pet your dog?"

We would wait, patiently, while every kid who wished to reach out and touch a big, friendly, panting dog could do so. Often a teacher, or a parent helper, would also come over, always smiling, always delighted to see the friendly dog make its slow way across the field.

But none of this works while walking alone. I walk down the street and no one says hello, no one smiles. We breeze by each other as if neither even exists. If I were to dare to walk slowly, and alone, across this same schoolyard at recess, there would probably be alarms sounding.

I have tried other solutions. The eldest daughter is, frankly, getting quite annoyed at being asked if she'd like to go for a walk. She makes jokes about getting the leash and making sure one of us carries a plastic bag, just in case. I have been watching other lone walkers and notice that some of them use props. One man, for example, heads into those same woods each day with a camera. I used to think it was to photograph the wildflowers or the fresh-fallen snow, which it is, but I suspect now it is also so that no one will presume he is up to no good.

I briefly considered walking one of the four cats— please don't ask how they ended up here—but if you cannot herd cats then surely they are also unwalkable. In good weather, of course, there is always the bicycle, and no one ever questions a lone rider. And once the snow falls and stays, there are cross-country skis to throw over a shoulder and snowshoes to tuck under an arm, even if one has no intention of ever using them. But at this time of year it is too cold for biking, too early for skiing, and often too icy and slushy for running, so there is really nothing to do each day but head out in the dying light and walk.

Alone. A suspicious character, up to no good. Someone who had better find another dog soon to walk him.

# Dog Wonder

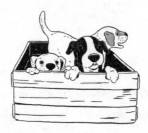

It had been a mild January. The sun felt like March, the wind like October, and yet the snow, knee-deep, was as white as it had been in the old days, before washed-out colour photography began tinting fresh-fallen snow blue and even yellow.

You could not help but notice this snow as it, too, had to do with unusual weather patterns for this part of the country. First there had been an ice storm, then a melt, then a great overnight dump of snow that stuck, like candy floss, to everything damp that it touched. Even hydro lines and eyebrows.

The kids called this puffed-up cotton-ball world magic. They said the woods were just as they are in *Narnia,* the movie version of C.S. Lewis's fabulous children's and adults' classic having just come out, and they were right. The fat snow was everywhere. It hung from the roofs and clung to the wires. It gave cars odd haircuts depending on how much drivers bothered to scrape off and sweep clear before driving away. It brought out the plows and the magic carpets and even the older walkers who would sometimes just stop at a corner and stare off into the distance, seeing a world they had not visited since childhood.

The growing puppy, Willow, and I went out, as usual, around noon for a long walk through Alice Wilson Woods, a park that covers several acres of hardwood forest, Precambrian Shield, and twisting, happenstance trails a couple of blocks from where we live. Only the evening before, someone on some television sitcom someone else was watching in another room had shouted out, with a note of incredulity, "Dogs can't tell time!" But they couldn't be more wrong. Dogs just don't read clocks—and likely because they have no need, as humans do, of external reminders. Fifteen minutes or so before noon, Willow comes into my office and begins annoyingly dropping a ball again and again and again on the hardwood floor.

Her predecessor, Bandit, a slightly larger dog, would come at exactly the same time and lay her big head on my knee, staring straight up until I folded down the laptop and declared the "w-a-l-k" about to begin. (Dogs, incidentally, *can* spell.) And the dog before Bandit, Bumps, would come in and pace about, her nails clicking on the floor, until I would cave.

All three never missed a deadline—which is more than can be said for their so-called master.

Off we went, Willow and I, hiking first along the unplowed back streets, then past the high school, then across the small park and in, through our personal entrance, to Alice Wilson Woods.

It was tough going, but I was not the first there. I had high boots on and still sank, at times, in over my knees.

Willow had, at times, to move through the snow the way porpoises will sometimes keep up with the prow of a fast boat, sailing free of the water, then vanishing into it, then sailing free again. When a powerful, energetic dog does it in powder on a day in which the sun turns flying snow to gold flecks and diamonds, it is just as wondrous to watch as porpoises.

We hiked through the lower half and then up a small rock bluff to an area I call the "plateau." It is flat and largely empty of trees here, apart from some thick sumac that turn the colour of dried blood in the fall and stay black-red much of the winter. There is open space here for marathon stick throwing and fetching sessions and there is even one part where, years ago, Bumps and I tromped out a new, original trail that is so rarely used even today we consider it our own private domain.

Except this day someone else had already been there. I have no idea who—the boot marks were more like fence-post holes than anything that would give away details about the lone early hiker—and I could see where he or she had stopped and scribbled something in the snow.

My first thought was a kid taking a shortcut through the woods to school, and presumed it was therefore either an obscenity, some currently popular cultural cliché, a paean to a rock band, or just the kid's name written in soft, new snow with the end of a mitten.

I went over to have a closer look and, for a moment, could not quite make out the words the way the sun was dancing and sparking on the snow. Yet when I moved to the side, and let the shadows created by the deep imprint of the mitten do their work, it was as clear as if a typewriter had been at a clean sheet of paper:

*Where the woods end, the fantasy begins*

I later spent hours on the internet trying to track down this quote. My first thought—hardly inspirational—was that it came from C.S. Lewis. It was impossible to stand in Alice Wilson Woods this late January day and not think you had entered some fabulous fairyland through a magical portal. There might not have been a wardrobe at the entrance to the woods, but the effect of leaving the streets and the park and stepping into a hardwood forest where every single tree was coated with thick snow was very much what little Lucy encountered when she first pushed her way through the heavy coats and found there was something magical beyond.

But I found nothing. And that, I must say, delighted me all the more. It meant—unless I am one day proven wrong—that the person who reached the plateau first that glorious day, the unknown person who stopped and simply could not resist bending over and saying something with the tip of his or her mitten, had reached some original inspiration in Alice Wilson Woods and felt compelled to record it, if not share it. For several days I would return at noon to the same spot. And though dozens of tracks formed over those days, no one ever rubbed out or disturbed the words. The mild weather merely shrank the snow until, a week later, the faded message looked like one of those secret notes we used to pass as children, writing on paper with lemon juice.

I know that person without knowing who it is. We come to walk here for different reasons; we come for the same reasons. I come here to walk with my dog—or dogs, over time—to lose myself, to walk and let my thoughts drift off until it feels as if there is no thinking being done at all. I do this deliberately, trusting in that curious multi-tasking machine—a machine that sometimes purrs along, often misses, once in a while stalls outright—that sits between my ears suddenly surprising me at the end of the noon-hour walk with an answer to whatever all-but-forgotten question was pressing at the beginning.

Willow comes to find herself. She comes to be as alert and focused as she will be at any time during her day. This walk is the highlight of a day that begins and ends with her being clipped to a lead and sent out into the backyard to do what needs to be done.

Here, she does what she wants, not what her ostensible master demands. Here, she is the master and the two-legged walker the server. He breaks off the dead branches that will serve as the daily sticks. He throws and throws again until either she tires of the game (unlikely) or he strategically fires it high into a tangled hawthorn where, with luck, it will hang suspended too high for her to leap up and grab and, eventually, she will give up.

Here is where she chases the squirrels that, uncannily, seem to delight in complicated physics experiments that calculate their relative speed, the dog's relative speed, the relative distance to the nearest tree, and the time available for safe arrival down to the closest microsecond. She has come so close their tails must tickle her snout; she has never come close at all.

I talk out loud while I am here. I imagine I sound a bit like one of those obnoxious travellers who walk about airport gates talking into their earpiece cellphones as if their business is, or should be, everyone's business. But I do it anyway, just as I suspect anyone who walks in isolated places with dogs talks aloud much of the time.

She pays me no attention. John Steinbeck always talked to his dogs, and in *Travels with Charley* would talk about everything under the sun—from travel plans to philosophy—with his big black poodle companion. Steinbeck was convinced that some of this habitual "doggerel" was sometimes getting through. "I've seen a look in dogs' eyes," he wrote, "a quickly vanishing look of amazed contempt, and I am convinced that basically dogs think humans are nuts."

I never see that. I'm more of the Dave Barry school of talking to your dog. "You can say any fool thing to a dog," the popular humour columnist once wrote, "and the dog will give you this look that says, 'My God, you're RIGHT! I NEVER would've thought of that!'" That is far more Willow and me.

We come to Alice Wilson Woods in all seasons, every single day I am home. We come in spring when the trilliums are so abundant it sometimes looks as if it has snowed along the bottom of the small rock bluff. We come in summer when the leaves are so thick on the maple, the elm, the butternut, the ironwood, and the ash that entering the small woods is much like stepping in through the flap of a huge cool, dark tent. We come in fall when the leaves turn and, despite the bright reds and oranges, there is a sadness to the air so sappy that it is a small wonder the leaves don't turn back green. And, of course, we come all through the winter, sometimes in winds so howling it seems even the dog has to walk backwards, sometimes on days like this past week, when the forest seems a stage setting for fantasy beginning.

We have seen wild turkeys and white-tailed deer. We were here one day as a black bear rambled through on its way to terrorize the local high school. We see songbirds and squirrels and rabbits and chipmunks. In winter she hears shrews and mice making their way through that busy subnivean world that exists between frozen earth and snow. We see fox tracks but only once have we caught sight of the fox, and it slipped in under the dark skirt of a spruce stand so quickly it was as if it had vaporized. We sometimes, but not that often, run into another human with a dog.

Willow is the third dog to roam these woods with me. The other two, Bumps and then Bandit, both eventually grew too old to come here, but in their prime all have been remarkably similar once they get here. Willow, mostly white with some browns, demands far more stick and fetch time. Bandit, mostly black with some white and a perfect drama/comedy split to her face, did the most sniffing and chasing. Bumps, black and brown with some white, who was already a mature dog when we moved here in the mid-1980s, was most content just to walk along, sometimes trailing, sometimes leading, almost always keeping to the trails.

All three had and have the traits of the famous sheepdogs with which they were and are somewhat related. When they crouch down, even in plain sight, they think they cannot be seen, much like an alligator in an everglades pond. When they stare at you, they think you know what they're asking you to do. They will attempt to round up anything available, from young children swimming off the end of the dock to squirrels racing for the lower branches of the nearest pine tree.

I know every single trail and every stone and every plant and tree in the woods—even the pool that forms each spring along the low-lying ground and seems to attract the same two rather dense mallards who set up house for a couple of weeks and then move on once the pool dries up—and yet I still get lost. This, of course, is intentional. I share the sentiment of American writer

Annie Dillard, who has a similar small suburban park she retreats to "not so much to learn how to live as, frankly, to forget about it."

I can, in fact, become so completely lost I forget how many times I have taken certain trails on a long hike. I remember once reading a biography of Charles Darwin and how, at Downe House, his country home south of London, he built a long trail—he called it "Sandwalk"— and would take to it daily for his "contemplative." So lost would Darwin become in his own thoughts and on his own trail that he invented a system for keeping track of how many "turns" he had taken, setting up a small pile of flint stones at a strategic point and flipping one over each time he passed. I have no such system, but the dog has flint stones she flips inside her head, because she always seems to know when we have completed our normal circuits and heads down the trail a bit in the opposite direction to the one I turn in, and here she crouches, stares back, and flattens her ears along her head as if trying to change her hairstyle to a ducktail.

One more turn? she seems to be begging. Just one more. Sometimes I give in; sometimes I do not give in.

We walked the entire trail system twice the Sunday that we discovered the secret message. It was heavy slogging and we were both, for once, tired when we made it back home. The date was January 29, 2006, and I mention it only because, as serendipity would have it, this snow-fallen day in Canada marks the moment year 4703 turns over to 4704 on the Chinese calendar. We have entered the Year of the Dog. The last one was twelve years ago, 1994, and twelve years before that, 1982. The next will not be until 2018.

The Chinese New Year begins with the new moon and the celebrations continue for fifteen days until the full moon is reached. It is a time of masks, lion dances, paper dragons, and fireworks, a time to mark the time of winter when, according to ancient Chinese legend, a beast named Nian would slink around the neighbourhoods, sneaking into homes at night and dining on small children as their parents slept. This is grounds for such a celebration?

Then again, perhaps the Year of the Dog is actually the year of the watchdog—though this particular dog named Willow will not much relate. She is afraid not only of her own shadow, but also of loud noises, other dogs, smaller ones even more so than larger, trash bins, plastic bags caught in trees, large lumps of snow and— remarkable as it sounds—fire hydrants. Mercifully, she is not a male.

Those born in the Year of the Dog tend to be honest and faithful, much as a dog is, with a strong sense of commitment and duty. They believe in justice. They are often opinionated and stubborn. They worry a great deal and are often too critical. In humans, those born under this sign tend to go into business or—so it is claimed—spy work.

I am from the Year of the Rat. The next one will be here shortly, in 2008. I looked up the characteristics and discovered that those born under this Chinese sign are charming, generous, but also quick-tempered and hypercritical. According to a thumbnail sketch I found on the internet, those born in the Year of the

Rat "make good writers, critics and publicists." I take issue with none of this.

The dog, however, was not born in the Year of the Dog. Because she is still a puppy of undetermined lineage and uncertain birthday, I can only assume she was born either at the beginning of the Year of the Rooster (early 2005) or at the tail end of the Year of the Monkey (late 2004). Those born under the sign of the Rooster are quick to decide, work hard, and are rather self-centred braggarts. They make good restaurateurs. I don't think so, though dining well is a prime concern for her.

Those born under the sign of the Monkey are considered very bright and tend to be extraordinarily successful. "Monkeys," the site tells me, "can run circles around other people with ease." Now we're getting somewhere. Monkeys are curious to the point of being nosy. They are clever, amusing, even sneaky. Those born in the Chinese Year of the Monkey, it is said, make excellent stock market traders, jewellers, and air traffic controllers....

SHORTLY BEFORE NOON the next day, she is in the office again, irritatingly bouncing a tennis ball up and down on the hardwood floor.

Bounce.

Bounce.

BOUNCE.

*BOUNCE!*

*BOUNCE!!*

"Okay, okay. We'll go."

And off we head again, off to Alice Wilson Woods to walk in the deep snow and chase sticks and come, once more, upon the fading message that the mitten left on the high plateau.

It is warmer now, and the squirrels are out, teasing her into chases that end, always, within a snapping finger—and jaw—of success. The squirrels move into the high branches, leaping from tree to tree, their condescending, sarcastic chatter driving poor Willow to distraction. She runs from tree trunk to tree trunk, jumping against them as if, somehow, this twenty-pound animal could fell a two-hundred-year-old tree. She barks and leaps, barks and runs and leaps and whines at the squirrels to come back down to earth—*I dare you.* A frustrated air traffic controller who is living proof that "where the woods end, fantasy begins."

And so long as there is a dog waiting patiently for its daily walk through these same woods, it will never end.

# ACKNOWLEDGMENTS

The author is grateful to *The Globe and Mail,* the *National Post,* and the *Ottawa Citizen* for indulging him during those moments when he chose to write about his dog rather than the state of the world. Thanks to *Cottage Life* magazine for placing the odd dog "Weekender" column on the back page, and to Natasha Daneman and Bruce Westwood at Westwood Creative Agency for their continuing advice and support. He is also indebted to Barbara Berson, his beloved editor at Penguin, for the idea of a book on dogs, and to lifelong friend Edie Van

Alstine, also a brilliant editor, for good counsel and strong advice. He is most grateful to Jason Schneider for his wonderful illustrations, to Karen Alliston for eagle-eyed copy editing as well as structural suggestions, and to Soapbox for their distinctive design. Thanks to Ellen, Kerry, Christine, Jocelyn, and Gordon for letting me tell some of these stories. Any mistakes, of course, are the responsibility of the dogs.